STRANGER IN THE VILLAGE *of* THE SICK

ALSO BY PAUL STOLLER

In Sorcery's Shadow [with Cheryl Olkes]
Fusion of the Worlds
The Taste of Ethnographic Things
The Cinematic Griot: The Ethnography of Jean Rouch
Embodying Colonial Memories
Sensuous Scholarship
Jaguar
Money Has No Smell

STRANGER
IN THE VILLAGE
of THE SICK

A Memoir of Cancer, Sorcery, and Healing

PAUL STOLLER

BEACON
150

BEACON PRESS
BOSTON

BEACON PRESS
25 Beacon Street
Boston, Massachusetts 02108-2892
www.beacon.org

Beacon Press books
are published under the auspices of
the Unitarian Universalist Association of Congregations.

07 06 05 04 03   8 7 6 5 4 3 2 1

This book is printed on acid-free paper that meets the
uncoated paper ANSI/NISO specifications for permanence as revised in 1992.

Text design by Isaac Tobin
Composition by Wilsted & Taylor Publishing Services

LIBRARY OF CONGRESS CATALOGING-IN-PUBLICATION DATA

Stoller, Paul.
Stranger in the village of the sick : a memoir of cancer, sorcery, and
healing / by Paul Stoller.
p. cm.
Includes bibliographical references and index.
ISBN 0-8070-7260-5 (cloth : alk. paper)
1. Stoller, Paul—Health. 2. Lymphoma—Patients—United
States—Biography. 3. Witchcraft—Niger. I. Title.

RC280.L9S76 2004
362.196′994—dc22

2003017995

Contents

STRANGER IN THE VILLAGE *of* THE SICK

CHAPTER ONE

Diagnosis

In March 2001 I learned that I had lymphoma, one of several kinds of blood cancer. Having enjoyed more than fifty years of good health, I was used to living my life in the village of the healthy, in which illness is a temporary nuisance that is quickly and completely cured. Cancer suddenly introduced me to the village of the sick, in which illness becomes a continuing condition for which there is usually no cure.[1] Learning that I had an incurable disease came as both a surprise and a shock. How could I have cancer? How much would I have to suffer? How long would I live?

These questions sank me into despondency. The menacing presence of malignant cells in my body ignited fires of fear. In a flash, cancer had abruptly taken control of my life and forced me onto a dreadful new path that promised unspeakable pain and endless suffering. The terrifying prospect of a slow and unbearable death made me tremble. These frightening thoughts quickly transformed me into a powerless person. I wanted my old life back, but in my dazed and confused state, I felt incapable of recapturing it.

Life-threatening circumstances, however, can sometimes steer your life in unanticipated directions. In my case, confronting cancer unexpectedly transported me back in time to the compound of Adamu Jenitongo, a well-known West African sorcerer to whom I had apprenticed myself as a young anthropologist. Lessons that I had learned twenty-five years earlier among the Songhay people of the Republic of Niger now took on startling new meaning. Somehow, cancer enhanced my perception and deepened my sensibilities. This disruptive new presence in my life made it possible for me to understand more fully that sorcery is first and foremost a set of prescriptions about how to cope with the vicissitudes of life. I gradually realized that this knowledge, which years ago had drifted into the background of my awareness, could make me strong. It could help me to confront the physical burdens of chemotherapy treatments and the emotional quandaries of remission with respectful humility and steadfast dignity.

As odd as it may seem, the unanticipated and devastating presence of cancer in my body opened a new pathway to personal growth and development. It deepened my spiritual beliefs, refocused my professional vision, and forced me to understand more realistically the symbiotic relationship between illness and health. In time, my experience of cancer toughened my body and strengthened my resolve.

Stranger in the Village of the Sick recounts this story of discovery, growth, and development. The pages are filled with narratives of my experiences in the worlds of sorcery and cancer, narratives about my life in the village of the healthy and the village of the sick. During my apprenticeship in Niger, I long ago grasped that one learns about sorcery through the body.[2] As a lymphoma patient in the United States, I soon realized that it is also through the body that one learns about illness. It may seem like a curious connection, but cancer and African sorcery, I have learned, share many similarities. In this book I use the lens of cancer to introduce readers to the world of Songhay sorcery, a body of practical wisdom that shows people—with or without illness—a way to carry themselves in the modern world.

Many books, of course, have been written about sorcery. Many of these have focused almost exclusively on the logic-bending feats of sorcerers who, like Carlos Castaneda's Don Juan Matus, possess knowledge "not yet known to us." These supernaturally oriented texts have made sorcery something that is usually viewed with either wide-eyed fascination or narrow-eyed skepticism.[3]

Sorcerers among the Songhay people of Niger do, in fact, possess knowledge not yet known to us. They are people capable of feats that, after twenty-five years of serious anthropological study and reflection, I have yet to completely comprehend. My book about Songhay sorcery, *In Sorcery's Shadow: A Memoir of Apprenticeship among the Songhay of Niger* (1987), was an attempt to demonstrate that sorcerers living in barren, windswept Songhay villages possessed powers—to heal and sicken—that defied our comprehension. I laced that book with stories of spells and counterspells, jealousy and betrayal. It was a portrait of an amoral world in which sorcerers challenge one another, often with lethal consequences, for sorcerous supremacy—the capacity to use one's will and skill to change behavior or repulse an enemy. In that book I hoped that readers would come to respect the incomprehensible power of sorcerers like Adamu Jenitongo, who taught me about Songhay sorcery over a period of seventeen years.

The experience of having been diagnosed with and undergone treatment for non-Hodgkin's lymphoma (NHL) has not diminished my awe of Adamu Jenitongo's sorcerous power. It has, however, increased my appreciation of the practical wisdom his life embodied. And so in *Stranger in the Village of the Sick,* I return to the world of sorcery and come to know the place, to quote T. S. Eliot, for the first time. Although *Stranger in the Village of the Sick* recounts many events from the Songhay world of sorcery, it extracts from them lessons that may well be helpful to cancer patients facing existential uncertainties and physical pain no less frightening than those faced in the world of sorcery. This account, though, is more than another story of a cancer patient who fights an insidious disease.[4] Instead, *Stranger in the Village of the Sick* is an attempt to use my experience of cancer to introduce readers to a body of pragmatic knowledge that can enable even the most physically compromised person to squeeze pleasure and happiness from an imperfect world.

❊ ❊ ❊

More than twenty years before I became a cancer patient, I stumbled into a world of sorcery. During an anthropological research mission that I conducted in the Republic of Niger in 1977, Mounmouni Kada, a distinguished sorcerer among the Songhay people, who lived in the village of Mehanna in western Niger, interpreted a series of signs that convinced him that he should teach me the ways of sorcery. I had been living in his village for several months and had visited him frequently. Shortly after my arrival in Mehanna, he had thrown divining shells; the configuration of the shells had indicated that I was a candidate for apprenticeship. When his son, Djibo Mounmouni, told him that two small birds, which had nested in the rafters of my mud-brick house, had shat on my head, he was beside himself with excitement. The marksmanship of the birds had confirmed what the shells had indicated.

"How wonderful," he told his son. "Another sign. We must initiate him as soon as possible."

My reaction to the birds differed greatly from that of Mounmouni Kada. Because I had been taught from childhood that a person's house should be neat and clean, one of my tasks was to sweep the floor of daily bird droppings. I certainly didn't consider bird shit in my hair a celestial sign. Besides, I had little desire to study sorcery among the Songhay. I had been sent to Niger to conduct dissertation research on the role of ritual languages in local politics.

Mounmouni Kada was a short, thin man well into his seventies. He had a hard face and eyes like fire. His seasoned determination proved stronger than my youthful resolve and he eventually convinced me to study with him. As a first step in this long and, as I was to find out, painfully dangerous process, Mounmouni Kada fed me *kusu*, a food that is believed among the Songhay to generate sorcerous power. *Kusu* consists of millet flour in which a Songhay sorcerer cooks pulverized plants that have been imbued with powerful ancestral words. After I had eaten my first batch of *kusu*, Mounmouni Kada told me that the "power of sorcery" had attached itself to my intestines. Witches, he said, could no longer look at me. Unprotected men and women would fear me. Despite my skeptical inclinations, I felt myself drawn to this strange new way of understanding the world. After my initiation, Djibo Mounmouni, a taller yet less imposing presence than his father, showed me how to mix sorcerous potions and how to recognize a witch. He also taught me sorcerous incantations and had me memorize the praise-poetry of the spirits of the Songhay people, who in the fifteenth century had controlled much of West Africa.

Djibo Mounmouni then urged me to visit his mentor, Adamu Jenitongo, a highly respected and feared sorcerer, who lived in another town, Tillaberi, which, like Mehanna, hugged the shoreline of the Niger River. Although I had met this man during my first stay in Niger between 1969 and 1971, I had not known of his reputed power. When I presented myself to him in 1977, though, he knew all about my research and my initiation in Mehanna. Adamu Jenitongo was a short, slender man in his nineties whose skin, which had long been exposed to the brutal African sun, had taken on the texture of cracked leather. He invited me to "sit" with him, a sign that he was willing to teach me about sorcery. By now I was eager to learn more. Adamu Jenitongo invited me to stay in his dunetop compound of conical straw huts at the edge of town—a location that overlooked

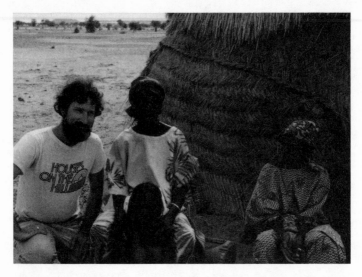

The author with Adamu Jenitongo's relatives in Tillaberi, Niger (1979).
Photo: Moussa Adamu

the barren emptiness of a treeless rock-strewn steppe that stretched like a moonscape to the east.

I sat, listened, and watched beside Adamu Jenitongo for several months. Everything about him was deliberate. He moved slowly. Before he spoke, he carefully considered his thoughts. He taught me incantations. I learned how to identify plants used both in healing and sorcery.

I emerged from this period of initiation confident—even cocky and foolish enough to try to practice what little I had learned. Before my return to the United States, an acquaintance asked me to perform an act of sorcery. He said that his employer, a French expatriate, had unjustly fired him and he wanted to teach the man a lesson. Thinking that a sorcerous action would bear no serious consequences, I performed a rite that was supposed to temporarily paralyze the man's face. Shortly thereafter, I left Niger and returned home.

During my next visit to West Africa, two years later, I saw this man again. He informed me that the sorcerous act I had performed, which involved the recitation of an incantation over the internal organ of a chicken, which was then buried under the threshold of the intended victim's house, had actually had results. The man's former employer had not himself been affected, according to my acquaintance, but the man's sister's face had become paralyzed, a condition that abated when she finally returned to France. Induced paralysis is a major weapon in the Songhay sorcerer's arsenal.

That same year I became temporarily paralyzed myself. I was on my second visit to Wanzerbé, the village of unrivaled Songhay power. I had wanted to go to Wanzerbé to meet Kassey, an inconspicuous grandmother who was reputed to be among the most powerful Songhay sorcerers. My friend Idrissa, who had been born in Wanzerbé and whose father was Kassey's husband, had agreed to accompany me on the trip. When we arrived in Wanzerbé, Idrissa's cousin informed us that Kassey had left town the week before and would be away for at least one month. Idrissa suggested that I visit Dunguri, one of Kassey's female associates.

After installing myself in the guest house of Idrissa's family's compound, which consisted of twenty mud-brick houses, I accompanied Idrissa down a sandy embankment to a road that ran through the middle of Wanzerbé. The space between the two parts of town contained empty market stalls. Just beyond the market stood a mosque with a minaret. We plodded along sandy paths between the low mud-brick walls of compounds, clusters of houses in which extended families lived. As we walked we greeted women who were pounding millet in their mortars. In the next neighborhood, called Sohanci, we encountered some of Idrissa's maternal relatives. According to custom, they greeted us and asked after our health. Next to a small neighborhood mosque was a clearing, in the center of which was a freestanding thatched canopy. A dozen older men, dressed in robes and turbans, reclined in the shade. We greeted them and asked after their health. Finally, we reached Dunguri's compound, which was squeezed between two large mud-brick granaries that looked like beehives and a corral for calves that had been fashioned from millet and cornstalks.

Performing the traditional greeting, Idrissa clapped three times outside the door of the woman's rectangular house. She came out, greeted him, and glanced at me. "Who is this stranger?" she asked Idrissa.

"I am Paul. I come from America," I interjected.

"Idrissa, come into my house. We will talk. Stranger, you, too, can come in."

We stepped down into Dunguri's house. Bright cotton blankets covered her whitewashed walls. She had draped a score of additional blankets over two beds that had been placed at either end of the rectangular room. She gave us metal folding chairs to sit on. She sat on a wooden stool and leaned forward, her hands on her knees.

Idrissa and Dunguri discussed the health and sickness of people they knew. So-and-so's son was in Niamey serving in the army. So-and-so's daughter had married and now lived in a neighboring village. Amadu had not been well. He had gone off to the regional hospital for medical attention, but the guinea worm still made him suffer. An older man had recently died from liver disease. Idrissa asked about the harvest.

"It was good. My husband worked hard and brought in three hundred bundles of millet."

"Our harvest in Mehanna," Idrissa commented, "was not good."

Dunguri nodded. "Some years are good. In other years the path is blocked."

Dunguri pointedly ignored me. For a Songhay, her behavior seemed completely out of character. Songhay people revere hospitality. They are especially curious about strangers. These characteristics seemed to have escaped Dunguri. I sat impatiently as they conversed, taking the opportunity to study her face. I would have never guessed that this small, plump woman was a sorcerer. Her puffy face did not look particularly intelligent, nor did her gaze seem forceful. Suddenly, I heard the word *stranger*. Dunguri had asked Idrissa about me. Idrissa outlined my work in Mehanna and Tillaberi. He told her that I wanted to write a book about sorcery and that I had been following the sorcerous path for more than two years.

She turned toward me. "Stranger," she said, "where did you get your rings? They're very beautiful."

Adamu Jenitongo had given me the rings, two fashioned from brass, one from copper, two years earlier. "They will protect you from those who want to send you sickness," he had informed me. "If someone asks you about them, say you got them at a market. Never reveal their real identity." I now heeded this warning. "Thank you," I told her. "I bought these rings last week at Ayoru market."

Dunguri addressed Idrissa again. "Show the stranger my granaries and animals. I have no more time to talk today." She stood up, stepped out of her house, and walked into the compound. Idrissa and I looked at one another. In all of my time in Niger, I had never been received so rudely.

That evening, after a meal of rice topped with a thin green gumbo sauce, I prepared for bed. I felt anxious and alone. As the kerosene lantern flickered, I slowly slipped into a fitful sleep.

Some time later I awoke to the tattoo of footsteps on the roof of the house. Was there a donkey on the roof above me? My anxiety returned instantly. I didn't move, and I heard nothing more. A chill wind, which suddenly swept into the hot, stuffy room where I had been sleeping, made me fear for my life. Fright compelled me to abandon the house to whatever hovered in the darkness. But when I tried to roll off my straw sleeping mat, I could not move my lower body. I pinched my thighs and felt nothing. My heart raced. Convinced now that some evil force had been sent to kill me, I was desperate to escape. What could I do? Thinking of Adamu Jenitongo's lessons, which seemed to fit these circumstances, I began to recite the *genji how*, an incantation he had taught me during the first year of my apprenticeship. Most Songhay people believe that the *genji how* protects a person by harmonizing the forces of the bush. For most Songhay, the bush is a place of powerfully destructive forces. If these forces are not brought into harmony through the *genji how*, they can be life threatening. Adamu Jenitongo said that if I ever felt danger, I should recite the incantation until I had conquered my fear. I now recited and recited and recited it until I began to feel a slight tingling in my hips. Encouraged, I continued with my recitation. The tingling spread down my thighs to my legs. My voice cracked, but I continued to recite. Slowly, the tingling spread from my legs to my feet. I pinched my thigh—it hurt. I pinched my leg and felt pain. Finally, I rolled off the mat and stood up. The presence seemed to have left the room. Completely exhausted, I lay down and fell into a deep sleep.

The next morning Idrissa woke me. I told him I wanted to visit Dunguri.

"I'll come with you."

I shook my head. "I need to go alone," I said.

I cannot explain why I felt obliged to confront Dunguri, for I was certain that she had precipitated the paralysis in my legs. The previous night I had responded to my fears like a sorcerer and, having weathered the event, I continued to feel like a sorcerer. I slowly walked out of Idrissa's relatives' compound. The morning sun pulsed low in the sky. The air felt cool and dry. I walked and eventually came to Dunguri's compound. Again fear overcame me. I then remembered what Adamu Jenitongo had taught me: "When a man on the path reaches the fork in the road, he must make his choice of direction and continue forward." With trembling arms and wobbling knees, I entered the compound and stood at its center, waiting. After what seemed like a very long time, she emerged from her house. She stared at me. Looking back at her, I tried to conceal my trepidation. She finally smiled and walked toward me. As she closed the distance between us, she even beamed. Stopping very close to me, she said: "Now I know that you are a man with a pure heart." She took my left hand and placed it in hers. "You are ready to learn. Come into my house and I will teach you."

❁ ❁ ❁

A number of colleagues tried to "explain" what had happened to me in Wanzerbé. Some of them said I had a bad dream, others suggested that I had taken mind-altering drugs, while still others thought I had an overactive imagination. I understood my paralysis differently. In Wanzerbé I had fallen into a physically vulnerable situation and had somehow found the strength to overcome my helplessness. Against the odds, a European emerged unscathed from a confrontation with a powerful Songhay sorcerer. This early experience in the Songhay world of sorcery contributed to my arrogance—especially about the impregnability of my body. Prior to my cancer diagnosis, I was ignorant about medical culture in the United States, knew little about medical procedures, attitudes, and behaviors, and had had only infrequent exposure to physicians. My health, in fact, had become a source of personal pride. I felt good about how well I took take care of myself, maintaining a low-fat diet, exercising regularly, and practicing yoga almost daily for more than thirty years. My favorite exercise was spinning; forty-five minutes of intense stationary cycling calibrated to lively music. In addition, I led a relatively stress-free life, had satisfying relationships, and enjoyed my work at a university in suburban Philadelphia. I even managed to find time to travel and write. In short, I liked my life.

Liking one's life, of course, does not make it carefree. I had professional disappointments: publishers would reject an article or book manuscript; foundations would turn down a grant proposal. A good friend or family member would experience illness or suffer a misfortune; and I struggled with minor health concerns, one year suffering from recurrent bouts of bronchitis. My physician, Brian Markson, said that I had developed asthma. For the first time in my life, I had to accustom myself to taking regular medication. I also had high cholesterol.

"You have a choice," my doctor said. "You can eat grass or take a little pill every day and not worry too much about cholesterol."

"I'll take the pill," I stated without equivocation.

By the time I was fifty I had established a minimalist medical routine. I took two puffs of Intal to control my asthma and one tablet of Pravachol to manage cholesterol. These conditions didn't limit my activities. I felt myself a middle-aged man "in control" of his life.

I scheduled yearly physicals. At each appointment, Brian Markson poked, prodded, and ordered blood tests that screened for heart disease, liver disease, kidney malfunction, and prostate cancer. Each year the blood work came back normal and he pronounced me in excellent health.

Several years ago I put off my annual physical, which I usually scheduled for the late spring. The summer and fall passed by without a thought about a checkup. I finally arranged an appointment, for a late afternoon in early February. As always, I expected to be in and out rather quickly, which would enable me to drive into Philadelphia with my friend Miriam to meet a mutual friend for dinner and a play. Miriam drove me to Brian Markson's office and waited in her car while I went in for what I expected to be a routine physical.

The waiting area was divided into a children's section featuring low chairs, benches, toys, and children's books, and an adult section that had been furnished with cushioned armchairs. Magazines had been neatly piled on corner tables. Shortly after I sat down, a pleasant gray-haired woman in a white uniform appeared in the narrow hallway that led to the examination rooms. She had my medical file.

"Mr. Stoller," she said, smiling warmly. "You can come back now." She asked me to read an eye chart and handed me a plastic cup for a urine sample. She eventually led me to a small examination room, where I sat down on a chair. "The doctor will be with you shortly," she said.

"That's what they all say," I responded jokingly.

"Really," she said. "He's not running late today. He'll be in to see you in just a few minutes."

Brian Markson walked in shortly afterward. He is a pleasant-looking, trim man in his early forties who projects a quiet confidence to his patients yet can admit what he doesn't know. I appreciated his humanism. He took as much time as needed with his patients; he genuinely seemed to care.

"How are you doing?" he asked.

"Well," I said.

"Today," he said, "I get to pick on you. Are you ready?"

"I always look forward to getting picked on."

He asked me questions about my regimen of food and exercise. He wondered if I might need special inoculations for travel I was planning.

"Do I need them for the Bronx?" I asked, trying to keep the conversation light.

He took my blood pressure. "One-seventeen over eighty," he announced. "You must be doing something right. Keep it up."

He checked my ears and throat and listened to my lungs. "Everything is clear. Why don't you get on the table?"

I sat on the edge of the table. Brian asked me to follow a little light with my eyes—neurological screening. He tapped my knee with a small hammer and asked me to lay back and loosen my trousers so that he could test me for hernia. I coughed several times. "That looks good," he said. He then began to palpate my abdomen, first the right side and then the left.

"Wait a minute," he said. "What's this?"

I froze. "What's what?"

"I feel something that shouldn't be there," he said. He took my hand and put my fingers on a spot on the left side of my abdomen and applied pressure. "Do you feel that?"

My fingers came up against something solid. "Yes."

He put my fingers on the opposite side of my abdomen and again pushed in. "Feel that?"

"Yes."

"Feels spongy, right?"

"Right," I said, suddenly wondering what could be wrong with me.

He moved my fingers again to the left side of my abdomen. "Feel the difference?"

"What is it?"

"I don't know," he admitted. "It could be that you have an enlarged spleen. It could be some minor intestinal obstruction. How are your bowels? Any constipation?"

I shook my head. "I feel great."

"You look great," he stated emphatically. "Except for this, you're in great health." "I don't know what to think," I said, feeling the blood drain from my face.

"Look," he said matter-of-factly, "as a doctor I find things every day that need to be checked out. Usually, it turns out to be nothing. I wouldn't worry too much about it now. It's important that we're thorough and follow up on this, that's all."

"I appreciate what you're saying, but I still feel as if someone hit me on the head with a sledgehammer."

"Let's get you in for a sonogram to get some idea of what's going on. I'll call the radiology department at the hospital and get you scheduled." He left the room, returning a few moments later. "The earliest appointment we could get is ten days from now," he said, frowning. "I'm sorry you have to wait so long."

"So am I," I said.

"Remember, these things usually turn out to be no big deal. I know it's difficult, but try to relax and not think too much about it. I'll see you again after the sonogram." He handed me his card. "If you have any questions in the meantime, call me."

"Thank you," I said as I left the examining room. I walked down the hallway, feeling very different from the relatively care-free person who had walked in moments earlier.

At the front desk, the nurse gave me several insurance forms. "Don't worry, Mr. Stoller," she said with genuine concern. "I'm sure you'll be okay."

I looked down at the forms. "Undefined mass" had been checked on the sonogram order. An hour earlier I had been un-aware of the presence of an "undefined mass" in my abdomen. Suddenly I could feel it moving inside of me. I visualized it, whatever it might be, slowly expanding. What would happen to it? What would happen to me? Isn't it amazing, I thought to my-self ruefully, how knowledge shapes our awareness of things—even things growing in our very own bodies!

Lost in these thoughts, I walked back to Miriam's car. She is a tall, willowy woman in her mid-forties with straight black hair and a warm, attractive, olive-skinned face. She had been read-ing, and was looking forward to eating at a small, highly recom-mended neighborhood restaurant in Philadelphia. Lost in her book, she did not hear me approach.

When I entered the car, Miriam turned and smiled. "Well, are you healthy?" she asked jokingly in her soft, smooth voice.

"Yes," I said. "He said that I was healthy, but felt a growth in my abdomen."

"A growth?" she repeated.

"Yes, a growth," I said numbly. "He put my fingers on it." I paused a moment. "I could feel it, Miriam. I can feel it now."

"How can it be?" she wondered. "You're in such good health. You have such stamina and you take good care of yourself."

"He said it could be my spleen or it might be an intestinal blockage, or maybe even a bad case of constipation."

"That's what it must be," she stated.

"I don't know," I said, suspecting that my condition was more serious than constipation.

She looked concerned. "Do you still want to go into Philadelphia?"

"Yes," I said. "I'm going to do what I usually do."

"Sounds like a good course of action," Miriam said. "Do you have to go in for tests?"

"A sonogram, but I have to wait for ten days."

"Oh, for God's sake!"

"My sentiments exactly."

She started the car. "Try not to think about it too much. It's probably nothing," she added, echoing Brian Markson's words.

"Okay," I said, thinking that it wouldn't be easy to follow this advice. I hoped my condition would be "nothing serious." Despite these hopes, I feared that the "undefined mass" would turn out to be "something horrible."

As we drove into the city, I wondered what it was about the confrontation with serious illness that provoked avoidance. Miriam veered away from any discussion of my physical condition except to reiterate, "You're in such good health, I'm sure it's nothing."

These bromides are, I think, a necessary measure in dealing with the uncertainty of facing disease. No one wants to hear a friend or loved one suggest: "If they felt a growth, it must be a tumor, probably malignant." Few people would make such a proclamation. Many people, however, would silently draw this conclusion. Uncertain medical findings cast the shadow of illness over personal interaction, clouding conversations and concealing thoughts. "It's probably nothing," your friends, colleagues, and loved ones tell you, "but it's best to be sure."

As the patient, you gratefully accept these reassurances, but cannot erase doubt from your mind. "He thought that my spleen was enlarged." I couldn't help repeating this to Miriam.

"He also said that you could simply be constipated. Why not think about that explanation?"

"Good suggestion," I said, trying to stay optimistic.

As we joined a colleague and ordered wine, we made a toast to our health. For me, this toast had suddenly taken on a deeper meaning.

I did not bring up my inconclusive medical news. We discussed politics and our work. Every element for an enjoyable evening had been put in place: good food, good wine, and good conversation. And yet, the burden of possible illness weighed heavily on my shoulders. I made conversation, but continued to obsess about the "undefined mass" in my abdomen. Just hours earlier when I hadn't known about the alien presence in my body, life seemed relatively carefree. How quickly everything had changed.

Despite these disturbing thoughts, I managed to have a reasonably pleasant evening. But home in bed that night, I tossed and turned. Would I have to have surgery? If so, what would happen to my classes at the university? Would I be able to continue my research? How would my illness, whatever it might be, change the nature of my relationships? Unable to fall asleep, I went to my study, turned on the computer, and logged on to WebMD. I typed "spleen" into the search box and read with great anxiety the connection between a symptom like an enlarged spleen and a variety of medical conditions, some of them incurable.

The next day was the first day of a new life—the life of a person stuck for nine days on the threshold of a new life. I didn't like what I saw beyond the threshold, but I couldn't dislodge myself. After the sonogram I would know more. I hoped that I'd be able to deal with the problem quickly and without too much pain. Then I'd be able to return to the relatively carefree days of my old life.

❊ ❊ ❊

From my vantage on the threshold of the village of the sick I wondered why my brief confrontation with paralysis years earlier had not made me more realistic about and respectful of illness. Back then I felt that if I could use sorcery to stand up to the powerful Dunguri, I could use it to conquer illness and even challenge death.

Once I had confronted Dunguri and earned her respect, I had no desire to study with her. I wanted to return to Tillaberi as quickly as possible to recount my experiences to Adamu Jenitongo. The news pleased my mentor. He said that the sorcery I had performed on behalf of the disgruntled employee meant that I had learned my lessons well and that the *kusu* had thoroughly attached itself to my intestines. He also said that the episode of paralysis had propelled me more deeply into the world of Songhay sorcery.

For Songhay practitioners, sorcery, I realized, is not merely a set of beliefs, as many scholars would have it. Instead, sorcery carries with it real consequences—bodily consequences.[5] Songhay sorcerers "eat" and are "eaten." "Are you full [of *kusu*]?" "How much do you know?" These questions are answered when a rival tests a fellow sorcerer through an attack. If sorcerers resist attacks through whatever means, they become stronger and their attackers become respectful of them. If sorcerers become sick, their rivals have bettered them: they have won and have demonstrated their superior knowledge and power. The marks of these battles are not only inscribed in the sorcerer's consciousness, but are worn in and on the body. Sorcerers may walk with a limp. Their arms may be impaired. They may become blind. Their betrothed might die before their marriages are consummated. Their children might die young. In the Songhay world, sorcerers must be tough because their actions exact a high price. I had learned, or so I thought, how to be tough.

My victory over a Wanzerbé sorcerer, however, produced mixed blessings. It made me feel invincible, a state which, years later, would make it more difficult for me to come to terms with the lymphoma cells that my body had unexpectedly produced. How could my toughened body have produced lymphoma cells?

News of my "victory" over Dunguri, which spread rapidly through the bush, had also attracted new rivals who wanted to use me to advance their sorcerous reputations.

Because I was now an apprentice on "the path of power," Adamu Jenitongo gave me additional rings, bracelets, and belts that had "drunk" the powerful blood of sacrificial animals. These power objects, like the sorcerer's body, must be fed with food and drink. He told me to wear these rings on the third finger of my left hand, the bracelets on my left wrist, the belts around my waist. He said that this "medicine" would work if and only if it "touched" my body, completing, as it were, the embodied circuit of power. I gratefully accepted these objects and wore them. The sorcerous comprehension of the world so fascinated me that I continued to study it when I returned to the United States to teach anthropology. I spent much time reading about and reflecting on sorcery. I especially wanted to know more about how magical words could protect a person from illness and misfortune.

In 1984 Adamu Jenitongo thought that it was time for me to return to Wanzerbé, which in the intervening years had become for me a space of fear. Sensing my trepidation, he convinced me that I was ready to face my fate. With reluctance, I traveled to the Songhay village of sorcerers, where I hoped to talk with the notorious Kassey. After an arduous journey by dugout canoe across the Niger River and by truck across a trackless countryside of dunes, thorn trees, and dried-up water holes, I arrived late one night in Wanzerbé. My friend Idrissa, who had been living there for several years, invited me to stay with him.

The next day I tried to meet with Kassey, but was told that she had other business to attend to. I spent the day talking to Wanzerbé elders about the history of the village and its mythic association with sorcery. That evening Idrissa and I ate a tasty dinner of millet and peanut sauce. We then sat in the little courtyard outside his house. People stopped by to visit. Despite the pleasant conversation, I felt vaguely and increasingly sick. When I took a breath, pain coursed through my side. I again felt the anxiety and general uneasiness of my trip to Wanzerbé in 1979. What caused my discomfort? Was it sorcery, poison, or a fever? Our water came from an artesian well. The food? True, others—unseen—had prepared it. Did someone want to do me harm? Both my mind and my stomach churned.

At nightfall I grew progressively weaker, but resisted sleep. Thinking of my past experience with paralysis in Wanzerbé, I believed that sleep would place me in mortal danger. Instead I recited the *genji how*, hoping that I might be protected from potential rivals. By the time the cocks crowed, my efforts had exhausted me. Idrissa, who had spent the night with relatives, came by at daybreak and greeted me somberly. He, too, had forgone sleep. His two-year-old nephew had fallen ill and Idrissa had spent the night in a deathwatch; the young boy had eventually slipped away. Grieving neighbors wailed at the loss of such a young life.

Then I received the other news: Idrissa's maternal uncle had also died in the night. A storm had caught him in his field. He had taken refuge in his straw granary and died of a heart attack. One night and two deaths. I somehow felt responsible. Someone had sent death to me, I thought, and in warding it off I had diverted it elsewhere. Dread swept over me. I felt intestinal rumblings. I ran to the hole Idrissa had dug behind the guest house.

What emerged in my stool, a small white egg, the most serious manifestation of Songhay witchcraft, shocked me. Among the Songhay, the presence of a small white egg in the stool is usually a sign of impending death.

"I've got to get out of here!" I said to Idrissa when I returned. "There's a truck that's leaving soon," Idrissa answered. By now, he seemed eager to see me go.

"Please tell the driver that I want to go with him," I said. Attracted by the smell of death, a pack of vultures circled above a nearby cow that had suffered the same fate as Idrissa's nephew and uncle. In great haste I packed my things. Soon a procession of people accompanied me to the truck. The driver started the engine and we chugged up Surgumey, a mountain that overlooks Wanzerbé. At a safe distance and secure in the cab of the truck, I relaxed, having fled a world in which sorcery had almost destroyed me.

I have not been back to Wanzerbé. The town is, to paraphrase Wordsworth, too much with me.

❧ ❧ ❧

Standing at the gate to the village of the sick compelled me to relive the terror I had experienced in Wanzerbé. Like Wanzerbé, the wait for my sonogram was too much with me. In Wanzerbé my confrontation with mortality slowed the passage of time; it also made me more fully aware of my body. The ten days between my physical and the sonogram appointment also passed at an agonizingly slow pace. The "undefined mass" was with me physically, but more so psychologically. One night I lay in my bed and palpated my midsection. I could feel the mass. Curiosity led me to push too hard. The mass suddenly moved. Pain, both physical and emotional, coursed through my body.

The day of the sonogram appointment finally arrived. Like many days in the mild winter we were experiencing, this one was sunny, with a few puffy clouds and calm winds. By early afternoon, the day was warm and lovely. The sun shone brilliantly in a clear blue sky. I drove the short distance from my university office to the hospital, which was housed in a building that looked like a Spanish hacienda, with cream-colored exteriors and a red tile roof. I walked into the reception area and was directed back to radiology, a department hidden deep in the hospital. At first glance, everyone in radiology seemed sullen. When I approached the registration desk, the nurse frowned.

"I have an appointment for a sonogram," I stated brightly. Like many people, I somehow felt compelled to be cheery in hospital settings.

"Insurance card," the nurse stated blandly.

I gave her my card.

"Have a seat in the waiting room," she said.

"Will it be long?" I asked.

She shrugged. "Don't know."

I sat down in a rectangular room lined with rows of chairs that faced one another. A TV had been bolted to one wall and was tuned to an afternoon soap opera. Magazines had been piled on the various corner tables and coffee tables. There were no windows. A charming place, I thought, to learn about one's fate.

A large man in overalls, a red plaid flannel shirt, and a green baseball cap sat next to a woman dressed similarly.

"Don't know how damn long this x-ray is gonna take," the man muttered in frustration.

"It'll be soon, honey," the woman said in a soothing tone.

"I hope it ain't broken, that's all. I need to work."

"I'm sure it'll be okay," the woman responded.

Other people sat in silence, read magazines or books, or watched television. I found a copy of *Town and Country* and began to read an article about restoring early-nineteenth-century farmhouses.

Finally, I heard my name called. I walked up to a young

black-haired woman holding a folder. We shook hands. "Follow me," she said.

"I'm doing your sonogram," she explained as we walked down the hall. "Ever had one before?"

"No."

"It's very simple," she said with a smile.

"That's good," I said.

She led me to a dark narrow room with a bed. There was a swivel chair next to the bed and what I took to be the sonogram machine, a large black box with a screen.

"Okay, I'd like you to take off your shirt and lay down on your back."

I did as she asked.

"I want to put this jelly on you. I've warmed it up so it should be comfortable." She spread a clear substance across my abdomen. "Is that okay?" she asked.

I nodded.

"Okay, I'm going to push this instrument around your abdomen."

She passed a probe over my belly in small circular motions. I heard clicking. I wanted to see what had projected on the screen, but couldn't from my position on the bed. She pushed the instrument to the side of my stomach and then came back, again and again, to the left midportion of my abdomen. There, she circled the instrument around a particular spot.

"Can you feel that?" Her eyes focused on the area that she had pinpointed with the instrument.

"No."

"You mean to tell me you can't feel that?" she repeated.

"I can't feel anything," I said as fear began to rifle through my body.

She nodded. "Well, we're done." She wiped my abdomen with a warm cloth. "You can get dressed. The results will be sent to your doctor," she added as she left the room.

It took me a few moments to dress and compose myself. I put my hand on the questionable spot on my abdomen. What was growing in there? I wondered for the hundredth time.

When I stepped out of the sonogram room, the technician shook my hand. "Good luck," she said.

What did "good luck" mean? I wondered as I walked down the hospital's sunny corridor. I didn't want some technician wishing me good luck. I found it strange that notions of luck would be infused into the increasingly cold technological contours of scientific medicine. Perhaps luck defines the limits of medical practice. When all else fails, there is good luck. When a medical professional wishes you good luck, the results of your tests are probably not very good.

The next day I received a phone call from Brian Markson, who suggested that I make an appointment for that afternoon. When was the last time your physician phoned to suggest an appointment? He obviously had news, probably not good, to report.

Composing myself, I drove to his office. The receptionist smiled at me and ushered me into the examining room without delay. This process was also not something I was used to. In the past, I had always had to wait with other patients before being invited back to the examination room. The special attention, I reasoned, was also not a good sign.

A few moments later, Brian knocked on the door and entered the room. He extended his hand. "How are you doing?" he asked.

"Not too bad," I lied, shaking his hand.

"Are you being easy on yourself?" he said, taking a seat opposite mine.

"Right now, it's not easy to be easy on myself."

He nodded. "I can't argue with that." He opened the file he was holding. "I got a report from radiology . . ."

"And?" I prodded anxiously.

"They can't figure out what you've got." He paused a moment, glancing at the report. "They've ruled out your spleen."

"That's good," I said. "Isn't it?"

"Well, the problem with sonograms is that they have trouble with solid structures."

"Solid structures?"

"That's right."

"You mean tumors, don't you?"

"Possibly," he said. "It could be almost anything—even a bowel obstruction. We won't know anything more until you've had a CAT scan. That will give us an idea of what we're dealing with here."

"A CAT scan," I repeated, realizing that the hole I had fallen into was as deep as I had feared.

"I'd like you to have the test as soon as possible. I'd recommend Community Radiology Services. It's easier to schedule one there than at the hospital."

"How bad is it?"

"It's not bad. It doesn't take too long." Brian stood up. "If you have any questions give me a call." He took out another one of his cards and wrote a number on the back. "That's my home phone number. If you want to talk, feel free to call me at home."

"I appreciate that," I said, comforted by his support.

"Follow me out. I'll write up an order for the CAT scan. Try calling early in the morning."

"Like phoning for a tee time," I said.

He smiled. "Exactly." He gave me the form ordering a CAT scan. "Good luck," he said.

I nodded and left.

My strategy of calling early for a CAT scan time was effective. The technician, Julie, scheduled me for the following week. She asked me if I were allergic to any drugs or to latex. She inquired about whether I had a problem with iodine.

"Iodine?"

"They inject you with iodine to improve the resolution of the film."

"Oh," I said. "No, I don't think so."

"Do you have asthma?"

"Yes."

"Then you need to take prednisone the night before and the morning of the study."

"I see."

"You'll also need to fast the morning of the study, except for drinking two containers of barium."

"Morning cocktails?"

"If you keep them cold, they're not so bad," Julie said. "You can stop by Community Radiology Services the day before the procedure; they'll give you the barium and tell you what to do. Any other questions, Paul?"

"I don't think so," I muttered. My life suddenly seemed surreal—undefined masses, sonograms, CAT scans, barium cocktails, prednisone, iodine solutions, and possible tumors. It became increasingly difficult to remain safely detached from the disturbing swirl of life with a potentially serious illness.

"Great. We'll see you next week. Good luck."

Again the "good luck." And indeed, the prospect of a CAT scan made me feel like I'd need a good dose of it.

❀ ❀ ❀

In the world of Songhay sorcery, harsh realities obliterate notions of good luck. Luck plays no role on the path of power. In that world you try to anticipate threats to the body to protect yourself from illness and premature death. Thoughts of "good luck" prompted me to reflect about the trials and tribulations of my apprenticeship in sorcery.

Mindful of my confrontation with death on my previous trip to Niger, Adamu Jenitongo suggested upon my return to Niger that I concentrate exclusively on a more nonconfrontational pursuit—the path of plants. I eagerly studied the vast varieties of twigs, leaves, roots, and resins that sorcerers use to mix both medicinal and sorcerous potions. My increasing knowledge of Songhay sorcery and the intimacy of my relationship with Adamu Jenitongo, however, also triggered a palpable jealousy in his sons.

"Why not teach them?" I asked.

"They're too young," he responded. "I must wait until they are ready."

In 1987 Adamu Jenitongo, a man more than one hundred years of age, began to suffer the effects of advanced prostate cancer. His older son, Moussa, a tall, lean, and even-tempered man, took him to Niger's capital city, where a surgeon at the national hospital removed his prostate. A network of friends and colleagues paid for his postoperative medications. Immobilized by the advancing disease and reconciled to his fate, he remained in his compound. In the months that followed, an unending parade of friends, former clients, spirit-possession mediums, and fellow sorcerers visited to pay their respects. He began to reveal his most powerful secrets to Moussa. In late February of 1988 I heard that my teacher and longtime friend was, indeed, close to death. I quickly arranged a trip to Niger. Sadly, I arrived one day too late. Moussa, who would now take on the burden of sorcery in Tillaberi, walked me to Adamu Jenitongo's gravesite. According to custom, I picked up a stone, spoke to it from my heart, and laid it on top of his grave. Back at the dunetop compound, Moussa gave me rings and bracelets that his father had wanted passed on to me. "To wear these things," Moussa said, "is to be always connected to our father." He picked up a large copper ring. "Take this," he said, "and put it on the third finger of your left hand." I took the ring and added it to the others on my left middle finger. I continue to wear the ring to this day.

Later that year I returned to Tillaberi to help organize Adamu Jenitongo's *kuma*, a spirit-possession ceremony that ends the period of mourning for a spirit-possession priest or sorcerer. The *kuma* is usually celebrated forty days after a priest or sorcerer's death. In Adamu Jenitongo's case, Moussa, who spoke, moved, and acted with his father's careful deliberation, had postponed the ceremony until I could attend.

One day after my arrival a large group of people filed out into the bush east of Adamu Jenitongo's compound. At a crossroads in the bush, the space where the spirit and social worlds intersect, a sorcerer from the next village recited a series of incantations over a clay pot that had been filled with a mixture of water, pulverized tree barks, and perfumes. People wept loudly, remembering the passing of a great man. The sorcerer from the next town called us forward to present ourselves before the pot of purification. He gave Moru, Adamu Jenitongo's younger son, and me a container of the ablution. We walked into the bush, stripped, and washed from our bodies the filth of Adamu Jenitongo's death.

The Songhay believe that the death pollutes a mourner's body, making her or him sluggish, indecisive, and muddleheaded. If death is not cleansed from the body, it, like power, will consume people, making them chronically sick, driving them mad, or even killing them.

After we cleansed our bodies of the great sorcerer's death, we dressed and walked back to Adamu Jenitongo's compound. Men from the local spirit-possession troupe took out all of the deceased's personal objects and laid them on the sand in the middle of the compound. Holding a gourd filled with milk, the officiating sorcerer, dressed in a white tunic, stood stiffly over the objects—an assortment of metal staffs, clay pots, hatchets, antelope horns, sandals, and clothing. He took some milk into his mouth and began to spit it on them. He continued to spray the objects until he had emptied the gourd. This act expunged the objects of their filth. As the sun set in the west, the *kuma* came to an end.

In the darkness, Moussa, Moru, and I ate dinner. Moussa asked me to come back soon so I could help to complete their education.

"*Baba* taught us much before he died," he said, "but did not have time to teach us about myths and plants. He said that you would come back and teach us."

I told them that I would honor Adamu Jenitongo's request and come back as soon as I could.

Two years later I was able to return to Niger. At the beginning of my second week in the country I traveled from Niamey, the dusty and ever expanding capital city, to sleepy Tillaberi, 120 kilometers to the north. Having taken over his father's sorcerous burden, Moussa suggested that I needed fortification. He worried that my status as a sorcerer who knew many of his father's secrets would trigger jealousy in town and provoke a sorcerous attack. We sat in what had been his father's spirit hut, a small conical structure woven in straw. In the dimness, I saw that Moussa had carefully arranged the objects that had been cleansed during Adamu Jenitongo's *kuma.*

After we talked about myths and plants, Moussa took out several cloth satchels—all black and all fashioned from thin Chinese cotton. From them, he poured powders onto a piece of white cloth, creating a small yellow dune streaked with ribbons of black, red, and green. Using his thumb and middle finger, he distributed the mixture into a small clay pot, which he had filled with water. After he had recited the appropriate incantations, some of which I knew, he lit a small fire, placed the clay pot above it, and fanned the flames until the mixture boiled. Gradually he added millet flour and stirred the concoction until it thickened into a brownish green paste. Once this "food without sauce," as *kusu* is sometimes called, had cooled, I ate it.

My problems began the next day in Niamey: heavy legs and back pain, the symptoms of *weyna,* what the Songhay term a "hot" illness. I went to an herbalist, who gave me a powdered mixture of two roots that I was to prepare like an herbal tea. I drank three glasses of the bitter liquid and felt measurably better.

Two days later, still in Niamey, I was the front-seat passenger in a Renault that rear-ended a Mercedes whose driver had

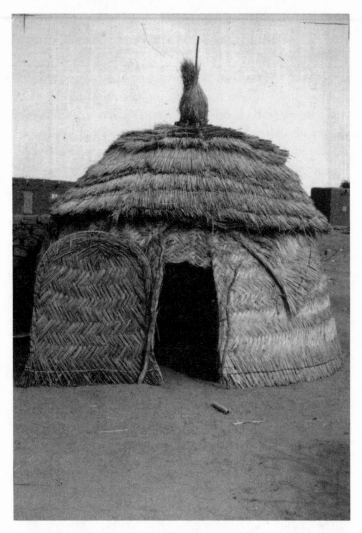

Adamu Jenitongo's spirit hut (1987). Photo: Paul Stoller

stopped suddenly in front of us to talk with a pedestrian. The impact accordion-pleated the front of the Renault and threw me against the padded sun visor, bruising my forehead.

The bruise had turned a deep blue by the time, the next evening, that I went to a wedding ceremony: cool night air, thumping talking drums, relentless praise-singing, all part of the bard's ritualized exhortation of gifts from attending dignitaries. I usually enjoyed these festivities, but on that night I felt tired and had a pounding headache. I recognized the onset of malaria. I wasn't too concerned. I'd simply give myself the "cure" as I had done on many occasions in years past. I dosed myself with chloroquine phosphate and went to bed, only to awaken in the middle of the night in a pool of sweat. My head throbbed. I felt a series of sharp pains streaking up my legs. In the morning I took more chloroquine tablets, but my condition didn't improve. By the next day my body seemed to be on fire. I took two more tablets. By noon my aching body was incandescent with fever. A visiting physician told me that I had contracted chloroquine-resistant malaria. She gave me three tablets of a different, stronger drug.

"That will break your fever," she said.

The remedy also broke my body. I remained in bed, my legs as heavy as water-soaked logs.

Days passed, but the fever, chills, and fever-induced hallucinations continued. I decided to leave Niger at once. The next day I arranged a flight to Paris and left the country two days later, exactly three weeks after I had arrived.

Had I returned home too hastily? Had I given up too easily? Before my departure, my Songhay friends presented me with a troubling interpretation of my illness. They suspected that I had been the victim of a sorcerous attack. They said invariably: When a person's path has been spoiled, he or she should return home.

Soumana Yacouba, a Niamey herbalist and sorcerer, said: "Your path has been spoiled. There are people here who wish you ill, but you didn't come to see me *before* you started your work. Adamu Jenitongo can no longer protect you from others. Next time you come, you'll come to my house as soon as you arrive. Go home and strengthen yourself." He gave me several satchels of plants to treat my condition. "Put these in hot water and drink three cups a day until you get better." He gave me a pouch filled with resins. "Burn these every day in a brazier. Let the aroma fill your house. The scent will fill your body with force."

I told a Nigerien social scientist of my experience. "Go home," he also said, "and gather your strength."

I spoke with an official of Niger's Ministry of Foreign Affairs. "Go home," he said. "Your path has been blocked, spoiled. You must go home and recuperate."

"Yes," I said weakly. "You're right."

"Your protector is no longer here," he continued, "and in the world of sorcery, people are always testing one another. Sorcerers are the offspring of fire; they can't contain their power. Go home and be more careful when you return. May God shame the person who sent this to you."

And so I returned home having learned through my body a fundamental lesson in Songhay sorcery: One must make careful preparations and be thoroughly protected before undertaking a task—especially with respect to the physical and psychological disruptions that a serious illness can trigger. My "illness" lingered for months: night sweats, shaky legs, dizziness. It was difficult to walk. I sought the counsel of tropical-medicine specialists. They harbored weak suspicions of falciparum malaria, the most virulent and lethal strain of the disease, but found no evidence of it in my blood. I knew better. I drank bitter teas and burned aromatic resins. Slowly, the fog lifted and I regained my equilibrium as well as my energy. I had learned the importance of preparation and caution.

❋ ❋ ❋

Having known the risks of being unprepared in the world of Songhay sorcery, I wanted to be ready for my first CAT scan. In this case, though, the preparations were not aimed at preventing illness or misfortune, which has a somewhat soothing effect, but at seeing what kind of insidious thing was growing inside of me, a much less reassuring reality.

On the day of the test, I awoke at six o'clock and took two twenty-milligram doses of prednisone, the queen of steroids. This widely prescribed drug not only opens bronchial passages but can give you energy, even a sense of euphoria, which, as I was to learn, can quickly turn to crabbiness. One hour later, I managed to drink the first container of chilled barium—not quite a chugalug beverage. I drove to my office, bringing the second barium container, which I drank as I stared at my computer screen. Fifteen minutes later Miriam picked me up and drove me to Community Radiology Services in a nearby town. Lost in our thoughts, we drove in silence along a narrow road until we got to a local shopping mall and a tangle of dust, construction, and traffic. We got through the main interchange and turned into a maze of low buildings, one of which housed the radiology offices. We walked into a square waiting room with cream-colored wallpaper. It was filled with patients awaiting x-rays, mammograms, sonograms, and, of course, CAT scans. A television monitor bolted to the wall displayed a video about health. I walked to the reception area at one end of the room and gave a woman the physician's order and my insurance card.

"Have you ever had a CAT scan before?" she asked.

"No."

"You've been fasting since last evening? And you've had the prescribed amount of barium this morning? And the prednisone?"

I nodded in response to each of these questions.

"Good," she responded. "Have a seat; one of the nurses will be with you soon."

Miriam and I sat down and stared at the television, which now featured a video on breast cancer. After a few tense moments, a young man wearing surgical scrubs appeared and called my name.

I stood up.

"I'm John," he said. "I'm a nurse and I'll be assisting with your scan today. Follow me back." Leaving Miriam in the waiting room, John and I pushed our way through the door into a brightly lit corridor flanked by dressing stations and dark, cold rooms that housed x-ray and mammogram machines. In the largest room at the very end of the corridor stood the CAT scanner: big, round, tan, and imposing. Like a tongue, a mechanical gantry emerged from the scanner's gaping mouth. John opened a curtain to a small changing room that had a locker. "Please put on this gown. Remove all your clothing except your underwear and socks; it gets cold in the CAT scan room. Make sure to remove any jewelry and use the locker to store your personal items. When you're ready, we'll go over the procedure."

I struggled with the gown, a less restrictive version of a straitjacket. Eager to get back to my "normal" life, I wanted to be done with the scan as soon as possible. I left the dressing room and looked at the monster that was soon to determine my fate. "It's not that bad, really," John said reassuringly.

"Looks pretty imposing."

"It's not as bad as the MRI."

"Right."

"Okay, first I need to get an IV going. We're going to give you iodine through the tube."

He tied a tourniquet around my left arm, tapped a few veins, tore the needle out of its sterile packaging, pricked me with it, and attached the IV connector. "Is that comfortable?"

"Not too bad," I said.

"Okay, before we begin." He paused a moment and looked at me directly. "Did you drink your barium this morning?"

I nodded.

"Good." He got up abruptly, went to a refrigerator, and poured a glass of opaque white liquid. "Have another."

"Thanks, John. That's really kind of you."

He laughed.

"Okay. So you've had your barium and you're premedicated with prednisone."

I nodded again.

"Are you allergic to latex?"

"No."

"Any problem with iodine?"

"No."

"We have to be careful with the iodine."

"Why is that?" I asked.

"An allergic reaction to it could be fatal."

"Oh, that's good to know, John."

"I'm required to inform you of the risks," he said with a brief smile. "If you feel any sense of swelling in your throat, let us know. There's a microphone inside the scanner. If you have any trouble breathing, inform us immediately. In the event that you have a negative reaction, we would administer adrenaline and—"

"Save my life?"

"Don't worry. It doesn't happen very often, but we have to be mindful of the risk."

"You mean that people usually don't die from CAT scans."

He chuckled. "That's right." He gave me a clipboard with a consent form on it. "This indicates that I've explained the risks to you and that you understand them. Once you've read and signed the form, we'll get started."

After the paperwork was done, John positioned me on the machine's gantry. He placed a hard pillow under my knees to support my back, then asked me to extend my hands and arms over my head. I felt as if I was being readied for the rack. "We do this in two cycles," he explained. "In the first cycle we take pictures without contrast. After we finish that, I'll be in to give you the iodine so that we can take pictures with contrast. Throughout the procedure, Julie, our technician, will be asking you to hold and release your breath."

John left the room and joined Julie in a dark narrow room behind protective glass. They pushed buttons and looked at monitors. Moments later, the CAT scan took me into its body. I heard the motor whining and groaning. The outer rim of its "mouth" seemed to move.

Julie said: "Breathe."

I did as I was told.

"Breathe." I was moved deeper into the CAT scan's body. "Okay, hold your breath until I say so, please."

Breathless, I was moved still deeper into the machine. A small yellow bulb beamed above me.

"Now breathe."

They inched me forward.

"Hold your breath, please."

They inched me forward once again.

"Breathe."

After twenty minutes of holding and letting out my breath, I heard John return to the scanner room. He moved beside me, near an opening in the machine. "We're halfway through," he said. "I'm going to start the IV." He took up a syringe filled with iodine. "Are you ready?"

As he prepared to insert the needle into the IV line, I couldn't stop thinking about my throat swelling up like a balloon. I nodded.

I watched as he slowly pushed the iodine into the IV. It felt warm as it entered my bloodstream. I tasted metal in my mouth and felt the iodine slowly shudder its way through my abdomen. My throat was dry, but it hadn't yet constricted. Maybe I'd get through this, after all?

"We're ready for the second cycle," John announced. "I'll be back when we're finished. Shouldn't take too long."

Meanwhile, my outstretched arms ached and I wondered if I'd be up to more breath work.

After what seemed an interminable twenty minutes, John again stood beside the machine. "All finished."

The gantry spit me out of the CAT scanner and I slowly sat up on it. "You did great."

"Thank you."

"Let me get you detached." He removed the IV needle and taped the insertion site. "Keep that on for several hours. It shouldn't bruise."

"Okay," I said, exhausted both physically and emotionally.

"Do you have any questions?"

I shook my head and headed for the dressing room. I wanted to get out into the fresh air as soon as possible.

"Good luck," John called out after I had dressed and waved to him from across the scanner room.

Several days later I returned to Brian Markson's office to get the results of the CAT scan. A young nurse with a pleasant smile led me immediately into an examination room. Once I was seated, she gave me a slip of white paper. I opened it and saw a name—Dr. Joel Rubin—under which was a telephone number. I stared at the piece of paper. Heaviness bolted me to the seat. The base of my spine throbbed.

"We made an appointment for you with Dr. Rubin," she stated very quietly. "It's for tomorrow."

I looked up at the woman, whose expression betrayed concern. "What kind of doctor is he?" I asked.

She cleared her throat. "He's an oncologist," she whispered. "I'm sorry."

In that moment the world that I had known completely crumbled. My head, suddenly heavy and weary, sunk to my chest. I stared at the floor unable to move. Cancer, I said to myself. How could I have cancer? I was tough. I had faced down sorcerers in West Africa. I had done all the right things: good diet, exercise, minimal stress. Would I be dead in six months?

Brian came in and patted me on the shoulder. "Sometimes I hate this job," he admitted. "You came in looking and feeling great, and I felt something that shouldn't have been there. And then this."

"I've got cancer?"

"It's very likely. You've got a seven-by-eight-centimeter tumor in your left midabdomen. Tumors in that area are almost always malignant."

"And Rubin?"

"He's a highly regarded, straight-talking oncologist. He'll be clear about what you can expect. I think you'd want to go to someone like him."

"What do you think I can expect?"

"That depends on what they find."

Another evasive answer, I thought. "Thank you for setting up the appointment," I said softly.

"He wants to see the CAT scan. Stop by Community Radiology before your appointment tomorrow and get your films. Once he sees the image of your tumor, he'll know the best way to proceed."

I nodded silently and got up to leave.

Brian put his hand on my shoulder. "It's not the end of the world. There are many effective treatments for cancer these days and Joel Rubin is an excellent physician. He and his colleagues are associated with the University of Pennsylvania health care system, which means he's informed about cutting-edge treatments. He'll work with you. Don't forget that you are in control of your own treatment. You'll be getting the best possible care."

"That's reassuring."

"I also know you. You have a strong will and you're in very good physical shape. I know this may not sound so good right now, but you're going in to this with many advantages."

I picked up my head and looked at Brian. "Thank you." I didn't feel very advantaged.

❆ ❆ ❆

Despite improvements in treatment and better rates of survival, a diagnosis of cancer is still perceived as a sentence to a slow and painful death. Most Americans don't like to think too much about death. Many of us can't even accept inevitable changes to our aging bodies, a sign that life is finite, let alone the specter of death. In the world of sorcery, however, illness is ever present in life. In that world, illness is a gateway to learning more about life. As for death, it is your continuous companion. The shadow of death often crosses the sorcerer's path. Despite the dangers presented by sorcery, many sorcerers live long lives. Adamu Jeni-tongo lived to be 106 years old.

During my apprenticeship in sorcery, temporary paralysis in Wanzerbé had triggered in me the fear of death. A potentially lethal "sickness" had prompted my evacuation from Niger. Anthropologists often face these fears in the course of conducting ethnographic fieldwork. Many fieldworkers in Africa have suffered from malarial attacks; some have been involved in automobile accidents. Even so, most of my Nigerien friends, scholars and farmers alike, believed that I had been the victim of a sorcerous attack, *sambeli*, for even if individuals have taken only a few steps on sorcery's path, as I had done years earlier, their bodies remain targets. Once sorcerers have eaten power, their bodies can be consumed by power.

In the practice of sorcery among Songhay people, *sambeli* is the act of sending fear or sickness to a victim. Sorcerers send fear by reciting the victim's name as they wind copper wire around certain objects. This rite is performed over a sorcerer's altar. Once the sorcerer has sent fear, the recipient's fright builds as he or she is gradually consumed by the sorcerer's power. In this way victims are humbled into a profound respect for the sorcerer's science, if not for the sorcerer himself.

Sickness is sent in an altogether different manner. A small

number of sorcerers possess a special bow and arrow that is associated with a particular spirit in the Songhay pantheon. On rare occasions, sorcerers take the bow and speak to the arrow—from their hearts. They then recite the name of their victim, usually a rival, and shoot the arrow, which carries sickness to its target. If the sorcerer's aim is good, victims feel a sharp pain in one of their legs, as if someone is pricking them with a knife. If victims are unprotected by magic rings or other amulets, the sickness will spread, resulting in partial paralysis and sometimes death. People who are well protected evade the arrow's path.

When Adamu Jenitongo took me into his confidence and made me a recipient of his secret knowledge, he thrust me into the Songhay world of sorcery. It can be an amoral world in which social rights and obligations are meaningless. The void created by this amorality is filled with power—of rival sorcerers, offspring of fire so brimming with force that they have little control over their spiteful tastes and desires. One step into the world of Songhay sorcery means that one joins an ever changing network of sorcerers, some of whom are allies who may become enemies, some of whom are enemies who may become allies, all of whom are rivals for power.

Moussa Adamu, after his father's death the principal sorcerer of Tillaberi, came to Niamey after I had been stricken with the illness that would precipitate my leaving Niger to tell me that local rivals had wanted to test his abilities by sending sickness to me. Although he was uncertain of the source of the *sambeli*, he was certain that the arrow of sickness had pierced my body. In Songhay terms, power had consumed my body. Someone had betrayed me. Someone had spoiled my path and I needed to return home. During the flight to Paris the central truths of sorcery became as clear as pure water. I realized that vulnerable bodies are consumed by the sensual world and that sickness can capture one's body and tie it into knots.

This brutal realization had forced my retreat from Niger. I feared that if I returned there, rivals might use sorcery to kill me. Although I maintained a safe distance from Niger for the next several years, I did not completely disengage from sorcery. I kept an altar in my house. I wore rings on the third finger of my left hand. Every Thursday and Sunday (days of the spirits) I recited incantations and poured libations—offerings to provide a measure of protection for friends and family. I performed these rites as a necessary obligation to the memory of Adamu Jenitongo. Fear, however, had displaced my passion for sorcery. I no longer struggled to understand the deep meanings of sorcerous texts or tried to comprehend the results of sorcerous acts.

During those years I thought often about Adamu Jenitongo. Sometimes he talked to me in dreams, telling me in his gentle voice that I had lost my way. In the dreams, I'd often visit him late in the afternoon, when the sun cast a deep golden glow on his dunetop compound. We'd sit on a palm-frond mat laid out on the sand near his spirit hut. I would talk to him about my irresolvable problems. He would listen intently as he packed grated kola nut under his lip. When I had finished, he'd say that my stubborn refusal to return to sorcery's path worried him. If I'd be willing to strengthen my connection to sorcery, he'd tell me, many of my problems would fade away. Despite his disappointment, Adamu Jenitongo would always say that circumstances would one day rekindle my passion for sorcery. Dismissing the importance of these dreams, I paid little attention to my former mentor's nocturnal ramblings. In the conscious world, I focused on more mundane, professional matters that steered me clear of sorcery's ambiguities. I read the works of urban sociologists and cultural geographers. I started a research project among West African traders in New York City. I wrote about sensory perception and West African immigrants in America.

❊ ❊ ❊

Now I faced a new challenge. Would Adamu Jenitongo be there to give me advice? As Miriam drove me to see Joel Rubin, I wondered if my new illness might be the result of a sorcerous act. Had a "rival" sent cancer to me? If so, should I return to Niger to seek a cure? Like a sorcerer's curse, cancer had suddenly and inexplicably appeared in my body. Could I expel it from my body the way a sorcerer expels a powerful spirit from a client's body? What would Adamu Jenitongo say?

It was a dull cloudy day in late February—gray light filtered through leafless trees. After signing for a large packet from Community Radiology Services, which contained the results of the CAT scan, we made our way to a branch office of Joel Rubin's group oncology practice. The weight and large size of the package surprised me. I pulled out one of the proofs and looked at myself, as it were, for the first time. I recognized some of my organs—heart, lungs, kidneys—but the more I looked the more anxious I became. I also looked at the radiologist's report. Brian Markson had stated the size of the tumor; the radiologist mentioned a "mesenteric mass, possibly lymphoma." Reading that possible diagnosis made me feel even more anxious and ill. I quickly put the report back into the package. Miriam patiently drove me to the next destination on an itinerary from hell.

"I read the radiologist's report," I told her in the car. "He thinks it could be lymphoma."

Miriam glanced at me with quiet concern.

"It's possible. Whatever it is, it's in my stomach and it's a pretty good size."

"I can't believe this is happening," she finally said.

Joel Rubin's branch office was located in a quaint eastern Pennsylvania town filled with Victorian- and Georgian-style homes. The building was in a two-story complex of offices fashioned from brick.

We parked the car next to a black Mercedes, a doctor's car perhaps, I thought somewhat bitterly, and walked up an open-air flight of stairs to the office: "Hematology-Oncology Services," the sign read. We walked into a dark, dank, and drab waiting room. The most prominent visual image was the picture of a smiling white-haired woman dressed in a housecoat. Above the photo a legend stated in bold print: End of Life Care. A pile of brochures lay neatly under the photo—no takers, perhaps.

I tugged the sleeve of Miriam's coat and pointed to the photo. Overloaded by the events of the recent past, she shrugged. I wondered if I had walked into a death space. Would I need end-of-life care? I had never thought about such a thing before.

From behind a desk, a young, casually dressed receptionist appeared. "Are you Paul?"

"Yes," I said shakily, trying to gather myself.

She handed me a clipboard. "Please fill out these forms. We'll need your insurance card as well."

"I'm getting tired of filling out so many damn forms," I said to Miriam.

"Just do it and try not to think about it," she replied.

When I gave the completed forms to the young woman, she smiled at me. "I'm Cheryl," she said. "Dr. Rubin will be with you in a moment."

A few minutes later Joel Rubin walked into the reception area. An attractive, big-boned man with a large square face framed by glasses, he wore dark dress slacks, a white shirt, and a striped tie. A stethoscope was draped around his neck. Soft green eyes offset an otherwise dynamic presence. I liked the contradictions that he presented. According to Brian Markson, he was a straight shooter, a feature that corresponded to his strong features. At the same time, he seemed like a person willing to express his vulnerability.

He greeted us warmly and shook our hands, and I followed

him back into a deserted corridor while Miriam remained in the waiting room. I noticed a large room in which recliners were flanked by trash bins fashioned from bright yellow plastic. A plastic sticker placed on the side of the bin read: CAUTION: OR-GANIC WASTE. Joel Rubin opened a door that led to a narrow examination room: two chairs, a swivel stool, an examination table, blood pressure machines, a cabinet with medical supplies and instruments.

I sat on a chair and Joel leaned against the edge of the ex-amination table and took my medical history, which, from the standpoint of medical science, had been relatively uneventful. My mother had suffered from clinical depression. My late father had suffered from bladder cancer, which was cured, and from kidney disease. Years in West Africa presented the most inter-esting aspect of my medical history. I had been treated for dysen-tery and malaria.

"You seem to be in good shape," Joel remarked, looking over my chart.

"I try to work out at my local YMCA."

"Sounds great." He looked over the history chart and signed it. "Why don't you have a seat on the examination table?"

I got up on the table. He took my blood pressure, which was high. "Just yesterday," I told him, "it was normal—one-twenty over eighty."

Joel nodded. "No one feels relaxed when they first come to see me."

What an understatement, I thought.

Joel listened to my lungs and heart with his stethoscope—all clear. He did a rectal exam—no prostate swelling—and took a specimen of stool—no occult blood. He tested for hernia and found healthy muscle. He pressed my lymph nodes and felt no swelling. "Why don't you lie back and unbutton your shirt?"

I did as I was told.

He palpated my abdomen, pressing deeply to feel the contours of the tumor. "I can feel it," he said. "You're in excellent shape, Paul," he observed, "which is a good thing. Okay, you can button your shirt. Would you like to see your CAT scan films?"

"Yes, I would."

"Why don't you get your friend and come back to my office."

Minutes later Miriam and I joined Joel Rubin in his office. He motioned for us to sit in the two chairs in front of his large desk. Behind him, I saw my insides displayed in two long lines of proof sheets attached to a backlit x-ray display case. He walked to one proof sheet and pointed to what looked like a nebula swirling in my abdomen.

"Is that it?"

"Yes. Looks like a slow grower." He gestured for me to come closer.

"Does it cover that entire area?" I asked.

"It's probably the size of a small grapefruit."

I gulped. I preferred to think of it as seven-by-eight centimeters. The radiologist had encircled the mass with red pencil. It practically filled an entire section of my abdomen.

Joel pointed to one part of the image. "You see here, it's wrapped itself around the bowel, and it's close to your aorta."

My heart raced. "My aorta?" I wanted to change the subject. "You said it was a slow grower. How long has it been growing?"

"Probably years. But I can't be sure."

"What's the next step?" Miriam asked.

Joel shrugged. "We know you have a tumor that hasn't brought on any symptoms. We have to find out what it is. Usually this kind of tumor is malignant, but we won't be certain until we get a tissue sample and have it analyzed. Once we know what kind of cells compose the tumor, we can take steps to treat it."

"How do you get a tissue sample?"

"We'll do a biopsy. Because the tumor is so close to your bowel, it will have to be a CAT scan–guided biopsy. They'll use the scan images to draw a surface matrix on your abdomen. Then they'll be able to extract the tissue from the tumor without nicking the bowel."

"We wouldn't want to do that, would we?"

Joel ignored my sarcasm. "The procedure is painless. I'm going to talk to a radiologist at the hospital to see if we can get you scheduled." He picked up the phone, dialed, and proceeded to have a conversation in doctor talk, only some of which I could understand. He described the tumor's size and position. "I'm hoping for lymphoma," he said before hanging up.

Listening to this exchange made me realize just how profoundly my world had changed in a few weeks. Several weeks earlier, I worried about how many calories I could burn off during a workout or whether I would receive a book contract in the coming weeks. Like Joel Rubin, I was now hoping that I had less deadly rather than more deadly cancer cells, something I would not have dreamed possible just a few weeks earlier. I worried that my life experiences, even my apprenticeship in sorcery, had not prepared me for the grim reality found along the pathways of the village of the sick.

"What does Paul have?" Miriam asked Joel, trying to get a more direct answer.

He took a deep breath. "We just don't know right now. If it is lymphoma, it could be one of twenty varieties. Each one indicates different treatment options." He took another deep breath. "I wish I could tell you more."

"Are some kinds of lymphoma better than others?" Miriam asked.

"Yes, but none of it's good."

The phone on his desk rang and Joel answered. "That's good," he said after a short call. He hung up and looked at us. "Your biopsy is scheduled for next week. Take the film over to the radiology department at the hospital and give it to Jim Rosen, one of the radiologists there. Don't give it to anyone else," he added for reasons of his own.

As we left Joel Rubin's office, I was numbed and overwhelmed by what I had to look forward to.

CAT-scan film in hand, we drove to the local hospital. Having already meandered the hospital's corridors, some wide and sun-drenched, others narrow, dark, and foreboding, in search of the sonogram room, I knew where to go. We walked up the steps to the entrance and crossed a wide covered driveway. Two young Asian-American men offered people rides to their parked cars. We made our way through the maze of halls to a radiology department devoid of people. Finally we found a woman working in the radiology record room. We tried to get her attention by tapping on the glass that separated record room from corridor. Vigorously chewing gum, she approached us. She frowned as she looked at the film envelope I carried.

"I'm looking for Jim Rosen."

"You can give that film to me."

"I was told to give it to Jim Rosen."

She shrugged her shoulders. "Whatever." She picked up the phone.

A few moments later Jim Rosen appeared. He was tall and dark and dressed in blue surgical scrubs—a garb that in recent weeks I had seen far too often.

"Joel Rubin said I should give this film to you," I said, handing him the folder.

"Oh yes," he said. "I've talked to Dr. Rubin about your tumor. Do you know about the procedure?"

"A little," I said, not certain how much more I wanted to know.

"It's quite straightforward—and painless. They'll get you into the CAT scan. The area where your tumor is located is pretty crowded."

"And you don't want to nick a bowel," I added, remembering my conversation with Joel Rubin.

He shuddered slightly. "Exactly," he said. "When they've

precisely pinpointed the tumor's location, they insert a hollow needle into it, and then put an extractor into the tube and clip off some tissue. You'll hear a click, but you won't feel any pain."

The description sent shivers down my spine. "No pain."

"No pain," he repeated. "They take the tissue sample and do a histological assay, which is—"

"A cellular analysis that determines what kind of cancer cells I've got," I said, interrupting him. During many sleepless nights, I had surfed the Internet to educate myself about the new direction of my life. "Will you do the procedure?"

"No. Dr. Stern will do it. She's very skillful." Jim Rosen glanced back toward his office. "Any other questions?"

"No. I appreciate your time," I told him.

"Good luck," he said.

"Why must they all say 'good luck'?" I muttered to myself.

One week later Miriam, who believed that it was important not to be alone when confronting a stressful diagnostic test, took me to the ambulatory care center of the hospital. We walked into a small waiting room. An elderly woman seated behind a small desk greeted us.

"Good morning," she said.

I presented my insurance card and filled out more forms and signed waivers, absolving the hospital of responsibility should some unexpected calamity befall me. She arranged the papers in a neat pile, stapled them, and smiled. "You can go over to the locker area and get changed into a hospital gown." She handed me a plastic bracelet with my name on it. "Put this on your wrist."

In the next room, an attendant gave me a key, a hospital gown, hospital slippers, and a cap. "What are you in for?" she asked.

"A CAT scan–guided biopsy," I stated blankly.

She shrugged and smiled. "Oh, those aren't so bad. They're painless. You'll be out of here in no time," she said. "Come back when you've changed," she said.

When I returned, Miriam laughed at my appearance: blue paper cap, formless gown that didn't cover my knobby knees, blue paper slippers, and an expression of confusion on my face. "I'm ready for the Hunt Cup Ball," I announced.

"Yes, you are," the attendant stated. "Have a seat in Waiting Room Four. You'll be called when they're ready for you." She patted me on the shoulder and muttered the inevitable "good luck."

We walked past a wood barrier that separated the ambulatory care nurse's station from a large square space one had to negotiate to find the various waiting rooms. Waiting Room 4 was situated down a narrow corridor at one end of the ambulatory care unit. In the narrow room of whitewashed cinderblock walls, there were two chairs, a television bolted above the doorjamb, and an examination table. The floor consisted of drab linoleum squares; the ceiling featured fluorescent lights surrounded by porous white soundproofing squares. Having been exposed to so many examination rooms, I began to wonder why they all looked like jail cells. Why couldn't they have windows, bright posters, anything to create a more pleasant atmosphere for those of us who had the misfortune of spending time in them?

Minutes after our arrival, a middle-aged woman introduced herself. "I'm Kathy, and I'll be your nurse. If I can do anything for you, just let me know." She asked the usual questions about diet and premedication. She had a confident, reassuring manner as she set up the IV.

"Am I going to get iodine?" I asked with no shortage of trepidation.

"No, they don't need to do a contrast with this procedure."

"Then why do I need the IV line in my arm?"

"They'll probably give you something to relax you when you're in the CAT scan."

"But they told me that the procedure is painless."

"Did they?" she said, looking surprised and shaking her head.

"Is it painful?" Miriam asked.

"There is some discomfort, but the tranquilizer helps. You'll appreciate it, it's quite nice."

I turned to Miriam. "I'm finally getting legal drugs."

Nurse Kathy smiled. "Enjoy them!"

"Under the circumstances, that's the least I can do," I responded.

The procedure had been scheduled for 10:00 A.M. After Nurse Kathy left, I looked at the clock in Waiting Room 4 and began an informal countdown. Although it was difficult to carry on a conversation, Miriam decided to wait with me. I didn't know what she might be thinking. I continued to ponder my radically transformed life. I wondered what the procedure would be like and what the tissue samples would reveal. Would the analysis bring with it a signed, sealed, and delivered death sentence? Would it, like the other diagnostic results, be inconclusive? My current circumstances had compelled me to spend quite a lot of time thinking about my life. Had it been a good life? Had I done what I wanted? Had I brought more joy than sorrow to family and friends? My thoughts made me both grateful and angry. I was grateful for my opportunities. I had lived many years in West Africa and met extraordinarily interesting people. I had been able to teach my passion—anthropology— and continue my research among West Africans. I had had the satisfaction of writing and publishing books. Most important, I had experienced much love in my life. But I felt like I was still young. There was so much left to do. I was not ready to die.

As these thoughts raced through my mind, the time for my assignation with destiny—ten o'clock—had long passed. Miriam looked at me and reached for my hand. "It's almost eleven. What's going on?"

"They always run behind," I suggested.

"I'm going to ask the nurse."

Minutes later she came back with Nurse Kathy.

"Guess what? They have not received paperwork from The

Cancer Center," she explained, referring to the main treatment facility of Joel Rubin's group practice.

"That's right," Nurse Kathy said. "They can't go ahead with the biopsy until they get the necessary paperwork from Rubin."

"Paperwork?" I asked.

"They need the results of the physical you had the other day," Nurse Kathy stated. "We've been phoning The Cancer Center to have them sent over."

"Meanwhile," Miriam said irritably, "Paul has to sit here, waiting."

"It's terrible," agreed Nurse Kathy. "I'll keep on trying to get them to fax over those notes."

"Thanks," I said, but I was angry. I felt like an object, a piece of baggage that had been misplaced. Sitting in Waiting Room 4 for hours dehumanized me. I had quickly learned the true meaning of the word *patient*. Considering medicine as an institutional system, "patients" must be "patient," for they have few rights and limited importance. In his highly acclaimed book about contemporary medical care, *The Wounded Storyteller*, Arthur Frank suggests that patients are subjects who are colonized by medicine.

> The modern experience of illness begins when popular experience is overtaken by technical expertise, including complex organizations of treatment. Folk no longer go to bed and die, cared for by family members and neighbors who have a talent for healing. Folk now go to paid professionals who reinterpret their pains as symptoms, using a specialized language that is unfamiliar and overwhelming. As patients, these folk accumulate entries on medical charts, which in most instances they are neither able nor allowed to read. (p. 5)

Waiting at the hospital for my CAT scan–guided biopsy, I felt very much like a colonized subject. No matter how strained my circumstances, I would have to wait and be patient.

❈ ❈ ❈

Given the realities of the American medical system, patients are often treated with insensitivity. It is also clear that physicians and other medical professionals are overtaxed. How many patients does a family physician, let alone an oncologist, see on any given day? A few minutes before each examination or consultation, the physician pulls your chart, quickly familiarizes herself or himself with its particulars, and then with varying degrees of skill, attempts to engage in a personal encounter. Ever conscious of time constraints, doctors are often forced to cut short their conversations with patients. Sometimes, important topics of discussion—for both physicians and patients—are bypassed.[6] In most cases, the patient is encouraged to be her or his own advocate. Don't be afraid to ask your doctor about new treatments or clinical trials. Don't be afraid to state your reservations about this or that therapy alternative. "Don't forget that you are," as Brian Markson had told me during one of our consultations, "in control of your own treatment." Well-informed patients receive better treatment. In the world of contemporary medicine, if you want satisfactory treatment, you have to be a strong advocate. This advocacy, of course, takes considerable energy, which you may or may not have.

Among the Songhay people, the relationship between healer and client works very differently. The healer is your advocate. He or she pays much attention to your being and serves as a guide through the thickets of the village of the sick. While residing in Adamu Jenitongo's compound, I once contracted a nasty gastrointestinal illness that made me miserable. To treat myself, I took some Western medicines.

"Could I see your medicines?" Adamu Jenitongo asked.

I gave him my tablets.

"This might be good for problems in your country, but our medicines might be better."

"I'll try anything."

He took my hand and led me into his conical spirit hut. "If you are feeling bad," he said, "the world is not right." He took out his divining shells and threw them in the sand. "Before I can give you plants, I need to set the world straight and then find a plant that is right for you. I will try to guide you back to health."

And he did. After consulting the shells, he asked me to give away a box of sugar to the children in the neighborhood. He also prescribed a tree bark, which I was to soak in hot water. Because Adamu Jenitongo's manner was kind and soft, I drank the decoction he prescribed with quiet confidence. I immediately felt tightness in my abdomen.

"That's the plant working," Adamu Jenitongo observed.

Several hours later, my ailment had disappeared. Through his care and advocacy, the world had been set straight.

❈ ❈ ❈

Responding to a much less personalized situation than I had experienced among the Songhay, Miriam finally ran out of patience. "This is so ridiculous. I'm going over to The Cancer Center to find out what's going on."

Twenty minutes after she left, the nurses received the missing papers and came to Waiting Room 4 to announce that the procedure was now scheduled for twelve o'clock noon.

Miriam returned several minutes before I was taken up to the CAT-scan room and told me of her heated encounter with staff regarding my medical file. "I asked the women behind the desk why it was taking so long for those notes to get sent over to the hospital. I asked them if they would like to be sitting in a narrow cell for hours, hungry and stressed, attached to an IV drip, waiting for something as serious as a biopsy. They looked rather embarrassed. I guess they didn't like hearing complaints in front of their patients."

"Whatever you said, it worked," I told her. "They got the papers twenty minutes after you left." The incident made me angry, though. I was being treated as if my time were of no consequence. I was grateful for Miriam's intervention. I realized that despite their isolation and psychological distress, patients sometimes needed to be impatient and demanding in order to be treated with a degree of dignity and respect in the medical system. As I lay there hungry, anxious, and tired, I wondered if I was up to the fight.

Finally Nurse Kathy came back to the waiting room. "We're just about ready. I apologize for the wait, but I hope everything will move smoothly now."

"When do you think he'll be finished?" Miriam asked. She seemed tired—ready to escape to the normal world for a short time.

"About two hours."

"I'll be back then to pick you up," she said as she squeezed my hand and left.

Soon after, an elderly man in blue hospital scrubs arrived with a gurney. I sat down and lay back and the man snapped the protective rail into the up position. He pushed me through the hospital's basement corridors as I looked up at a network of pipes. For some reason, the ceiling seemed to be curved, which made the corridors more like tunnels than hallways. In my state, I felt like I was being pushed through a large intestine. After several turns, a descent down a ramp and an ascent up an elevator, we finally arrived at CAT scan. The man parked me in a hallway. In the distance, I could hear the familiar whir of the scanner. Apparently, I'd have to wait a bit longer.

Two nurses appeared after a few moments. They again apologized for the delay and peppered me with questions about my allergies and other medical conditions.

"What are you having done today?" one of them asked.

"They need to take a biopsy of a mass in my abdomen. It

could be a bowel obstruction," I added, giving voice to wishful thinking.

"Could be," one of them replied skeptically.

The attending radiologist walked in just as the nurses had finished their interview. "Good day, Mr. Stoller. I'm Dr. Stern. How are you today?"

"I'm a little nervous," I admitted.

"We'll give you something to calm you down once we get going." A white laboratory coat offset her dark hair and olive complexion. Her comportment inspired confidence; besides that, I had cousins whose name was Stern. "So we're going to get some tissue from the mass in the abdomen?"

"That's right," I said.

"Did anyone put a scope down your throat to look at your bowel?"

"No," I answered, bewildered by her question.

She shook her head. "I can't believe," she said to the nurses, and perhaps to me, "that they didn't look to see if there was bowel involvement. The tumor is so close to the bowel."

This comment, as one might imagine, did not have a calming effect. Could they be wrong? I wondered. I desperately wanted to have confidence in the abilities of my physicians and in the diagnostic procedures they employed. If I felt that I was in competent hands, I might be able to deal with the "undefined mass" growing inside of me.

※ ※ ※

What is it about our medical system that provokes a crisis of confidence? American medicine is the envy of the world. Medical science has advanced in leaps and bounds in the past few decades. Sophisticated imaging technologies like CAT, PET, and MRI scans have increased diagnostic precision.[7] New surgical techniques have not only improved the patient's quality of life, but have extended her or his life expectancy. Expanding knowledge of human genetics has produced new anticancer drugs like Gleevec and Herceptin that extend and improve the lives of cancer patients.[8] Men and women with cancer are able to live longer and fuller lives.

Perhaps part of the problem lies in how medical specialists envision their profession. All of them are trained in science and employ the scientific method to diagnose and treat diseases. They use increasingly sophisticated and expensive technology to refine their diagnoses and treatments. Given the expense that a technologically sophisticated medicine entails, they have become increasingly entangled in medical institutions. Institutional demands—including extensive paperwork—increase the medical professional's patient load, meaning that there is less time for individual patients, who often get lost in the system.[9] Among the Songhay, the healer, who has the time and symbolic stature to inspire confidence, guides the client through the illness. The healer holds your hand and walks you through the twists and curves of the village of the sick. The healer attempts to set the world straight so that you might return to the village of the healthy.

❊ ❊ ❊

As I lay on the gurney in a hospital corridor outside the CAT-scan room, the world seemed hopelessly out of whack, a sense that my expression must have betrayed.

Karen Stern looked at me. "Are you okay, Mr. Stoller?"

I nodded.

"Do you have any questions about the procedure?"

"No."

"Good. We should get going in a few moments. Good luck."

I managed to walk into the CAT-scan room and get on the gantry, the narrow platform that transports the subject into the center of the machine. A nurse attached a pulse monitor clip to my right index finger. She also attached the sleeve of the blood-pressure machine. She smiled. "You've been in the CAT scan before?"

"Once."

"Well, this time you don't have to hold your breath and you won't be getting iodine."

The sight of wires and sleeves attached to my body at the precipice of a body-consuming machine was pretty unsettling.

The nurses joined Karen Stern behind the protective partition. The machine took my body into its innards. I looked up and saw a beam of light. The machine whirred. After a few moments, a nurse came in and coated my abdomen with a yellow-brown sterilizing fluid. She then lay a square matrix that looked like a checkerboard over my abdomen. Guided by the CAT-scan image of the tumor, Karen Stern isolated an entry point on my skin. Accompanied by the nurses, she came into the room and marked an *X* on my abdomen.

"How are you doing?" she asked.

"Fine." I was beginning to realize that it was easier to simply say "fine." This pleasant physician, I reasoned, did not have the time to listen to recitations of pain and anxiety.

"Would you like more tranquilizer?"

I did not want to admit my weakness. Being strong was a central part of my middle-class male socialization. What's more, my experience in the Songhay world of sorcery had conditioned me to be tough. "I'm okay."

"We are about ready," she said. "I'm going to insert a hollow needle into the tumor and then remove tissue samples. The click that you'll hear means that I gathered some samples and have removed them through the tube." She studied my facial expression.

"Are you ready?"

"Yes," I said.

She left and returned with biopsy instruments. She held the

hollow needle in her hand. "Okay, I'm going to insert the needle. Take a deep breath and hold it."

I took a deep breath and she stuck the needle into my abdomen. I felt a considerable amount of pain as the needle slowly entered what I took to be the tumor. "We're in," she said to the nurses. "How's his pressure?"

One of the nurses looked at the machine, which had been reading my blood pressure. "It's not working," she stated flatly.

"I'll do his pressure by hand," the other nurse said.

Meanwhile, I looked at the needle, which resembled a knife stuck in my gut. My pulse raced. The sleeve of the manual blood-pressure device tightened around my arm. Karen Stern stood next to me. "Excuse me," I said finally, "but I think I would like a little more of that tranquilizer."

"Give him twenty-five milligrams more," Karen Stern said.

My pulse slowed; blood pressure returned to normal. I looked at the hollow tube sticking out of my stomach and didn't care anymore. I noticed the watch Karen Stern wore on her wrist. "Would you like a new watch?" I asked. "I can get you a Rolex in New York for twenty bucks."

"Oh, really," she said. "I'd like that."

"Guaranteed for two weeks," I said, thinking about how far away I was from my field research on the streets of New York City.

She looked at the nurses. "I think we're ready." She looked at me. "I'm going to extract some tissue samples now," she said. She leaned over me and inserted an instrument into the tube. I heard a click. She then carefully put the tissue sample in a container. She extracted four small slices of the tumor.

"Is it over?" I asked, having failed in my attempt to divert my thoughts from the procedure.

"It is. You did great." She patted my shoulder. "I'm looking forward to the Rolex." She started to walk out. "The nurse will give you postoperative instructions. Good luck."

The nurses put a bandage on the entry point.

"You did great, Mr. Stoller," one of the nurses said. "They'll take the samples to pathology to determine what kind of cells are present."

I got off the CAT-scan gantry and staggered over to the transport gurney. A volunteer was waiting. "Ready to go?" he asked.

"Yes."

"We really enjoyed talking to you, Mr. Stoller," one of the nurses said. "Maybe I'll take one of your courses at the university."

"That would be great," I said as the volunteer took me back to Waiting Room 4.

❈ ❈ ❈

After the biopsy I struggled to resign myself to a life with cancer. My world had changed. Prior to the office visit with Brian Markson, I hadn't thought very much about my health. I hadn't pondered the possibility of a "premature" death. The members of my family generally lived long lives. Now, as the time between the CAT scan–guided biopsy and the laboratory results stretched into an interminable wait, I had come to a fork in the road. What kind of cancer cells did I have? Before this stretch of diagnostic procedures, I thought that I, like the men in my family, would enjoy good health well into my nineties. Now I wondered if I would survive one year, two years, perhaps five. Ten years suddenly seemed like a lifetime. If only I could have another ten years.

Like a character from Dostoyevsky's *The Brothers Karamazov*, I felt like a defendant in an existential trial. I had somehow violated some law, which meant that medical professionals felt compelled to gather evidence. At first the evidence had been inconclusive, which meant that they had to gather more data. At no time did these investigators, as in Dostoyevsky's philosophical thriller, reveal to me the full substance of their findings, let alone their thoughts and feelings about them. They remained tight-lipped, but did manage to say, "We need more information." As the defendant in this existential trial, my state of helplessness gradually gave way to numbness. Being numb made the trial easier to bear.

When sentencing day finally came, Miriam drove me to my appointment with Joel Rubin at The Cancer Center. My anxiety was overwhelming. I didn't notice my surroundings. Like a zombie, I signed in, sat down, and waited. Several minutes later, Joel Rubin came out to greet us. He then personally took my weight and blood pressure. Once he recorded those numbers, he asked us both to follow him back to an examination room. I felt like a dead man walking to the gas chamber. Once we were seated, Joel sat on a swivel chair, looked at me, and took a deep breath.

"Paul, you have cancer," he said softly. "Non-Hodgkin's lymphoma."

Even though I had expected such a pronouncement, the word *cancer* still shocked me.

"The bad news," Joel went on, "is that its cancer. The good news is that it appears to be a slow-growing lymphoma. Your tumor has been growing a long time."

"Can I see the lab report?" I asked.

He gave me two sheets. I glanced at a section marked "B-cell follicular lymphoma," a cancer of the blood cells that fight infection.

Miriam asked: "What's the prognosis?," a rather unencumbered way of asking how long I would live.

"We've made great progress in lymphoma treatments," Joel explained. He wrote down several Internet addresses. "I would recommend checking out these sites. They have a great deal of information on lymphoma. You should also look up the literature on Rituxan, which is a new antibody used to attack lymphoma cells. Rituxan has improved treatment responses." Joel seemed to think that information might be one way to deal with anxiety.

"But what about Paul?" Miriam asked again.

Joel leaned forward in his chair. "Given his age and physical condition, I would expect Paul to live for decades."

That began to make me feel a little better. "Will I need to get chemotherapy?"

"Yes. You can wait until the disease is symptomatic, if you like. You can get traditional chemotherapy drugs for lymphoma. Or you may want to opt for a newer treatment that combines Rituxan with the chemotherapy drugs. First, I'd like you to learn as much as you can about the available treatments and then we'll make an informed decision."

As he mentioned the awful inevitabilities that I would have to endure, I heard Adamu Jenitongo's soft voice. I hadn't heard that voice for a long time. As always, it came to me during pivotal moments. "Do not be afraid," he said. "No matter what happens, I'm still with you." The voice filled me with quiet confidence, but I wondered where it might lead me.

As Adamu Jenitongo's voice faded away, Joel pushed his chair a bit closer to us. "Before you can make a decision about treatment, we need to stage the disease."

"What does that mean?" I asked.

"Based on the CAT scan, we know that lymphoma cells have not spread to your lungs, and the physical exam indicates that your peripheral lymph nodes are normal. But we do need to know if the bone marrow is involved."

"How do you do that?"

"A bone marrow biopsy," Joel said. "And if it's okay with you, we'd like to do that today."

"What does that entail?" I asked, fearing the worst. I had hoped to have a short respite from diagnostic tests.

"It's not too bad. I've had patients get them and go off and play sports."

"But what does it entail?" I asked again.

"After numbing the back of your pelvis, I'll stick a needle into the bone and extract bone marrow samples. You shouldn't feel anything, except for a little pain when I aspirate the marrow."

"That doesn't sound like fun, but let's get on with it." I wanted to get this over with as soon as possible.

"Miriam," he said, "you can stay if you like."

"No. I'll wait outside," she said.

When she had left the room, I looked at Joel. "You know, this has hit me like a hammer. Here I am in full stride. I'm writing, teaching, and traveling. I enjoy my life, I feel well, and now I have to confront cancer."

"Well," Joel said sympathetically, "let's try to get you into remission. There's no reason why you can't lead a full life. You'll have to manage your lymphoma forever, but it *can* be managed." He stood up. "I'll go and get the nurse."

A few moments later Joel came back with the nurse, who carried a tray of test tubes and microscope slides. Joel put on latex gloves. The nurse helped him into a surgical gown.

"Okay, Paul, I'd like you to lay facedown on the table and loosen your pants."

I lay there with my backside exposed, feeling even more vulnerable.

"First I'm going to swab you with this sterile fluid."

I felt the fluid spread over the small of my back like a cool, soft wave.

"Now," Joel said softly, "I'm going to inject novocaine into the pelvic bone. It will hurt a bit at first."

Joel was true to his word. The pain made me wince. "You weren't kidding." I said.

Joel moved an instrument around my pelvic bone. "Okay, I'm going to aspirate now. This is going to hurt, but just for a moment."

As I heard the sucking noise, the pain, though of short duration, took my breath away.

I made it through the rest of the biopsy by simply gritting my teeth and hoping that it would end quickly. Unfortunately, the procedure had to be repeated on the other side of my hip. Finally, Joel looked over the quality of his samples and said, "I think we've got enough. We're finished." I heard tape being drawn and cut. "I'm going to get you bandaged up and you'll be ready to go."

I managed to pull up my jeans and roll off the examination table.

"You shouldn't shower for twenty-four hours," Joel instructed me. "Make sure to change the bandage every day. Don't take a bath. If the insertion site becomes red, call me. That's not likely, though. We'll have the results of the biopsy shortly. Call me for the results and come back in one month to begin your treatment."

"Thank you," I said as I walked stiffly to the door. The agonizing diagnostic trial had ended and a verdict had been rendered. I had an incurable disease, but at least now I knew that my death was probably not imminent. I had officially become a cancer patient.

❀ ❀ ❀

Being thrust into a new world that would change my life forever prompted me to think long and hard about my experience among the Songhay people of the Republic of Niger. I thought not only about my experiences as an apprentice to Songhay sorcerers, but also about how differently Americans and Songhay people experience the world. One great difference is how Americans and Songhay reckon time. I relived endless rides on public transportation through the Nigerien countryside. As a young anthropologist, I often took *le rapide,* usually a sputtering bus that would chug up the slope of a mesa. Overloaded and burdened with worn brake pads, it would dangerously race down the slope. You never knew what would happen when you took *le rapide*. You could be certain, though, of two things: there would be frequent stops along the way and the trip would take longer than expected. Drivers would stop, of course, to pick up passengers. In the afternoons, they would stop to recite obligatory Muslim prayers. If it was market day in a particular village, they might stop there. Sometimes they would stop to repair a flat tire—always a possibility on dirt roads where sharp acacia thorns had fallen from the trees bordering the highway. Sometimes drivers would run out of gas, which could cause very long delays.

At first I found it difficult to adjust to these circumstances. Like most Americans, I wanted a trip to be speedy. If I boarded a bus, I wanted to arrive at the destination "on time." In fact, I would choose public carriers, airlines mostly, that, according to travel experts, had a high percentage of on-time arrivals. This informed choice created a sense of certainty. If I chose airline X it was almost certain that I'd be on time. Feeling confident about the outcomes of our choices gives us a sense of control over our lives—something that most Americans strive for.

Most Songhay people see the world quite differently. They believe that they have little control over what happens to them. Many of them follow a fatalistic path in which uncertainty, rather than certainty, governs their journey through life. Most Songhay people never know what to expect when they board *le rapide*. Many people I got to know in Niger, in fact, exhibit what the philosopher John Dewey, in *The Quest for Certainty* (1929), called negative capability—the rare quality of being able to live with ambiguous uncertainty.

Like many Americans, I have a difficult time dealing with ambiguous uncertainty. In our mainstream culture, we prefer quick, clear, concrete answers to difficult questions. We'd like to believe that we are able to control our destiny. We expect our flights to be on time. If we get sick, we expect a quick fix. What better way to treat illness than to take a course of antibiotics and get better? How many of us are able or willing to jump into a fast-moving stream and let the current carry us to an uncertain destination? Most of us would feel that we were being foolhardy if we did so.

The process of diagnosis, of course, erases certainty from a person's life. The possibility of serious illness involuntarily throws you into a fast-moving stream, the current of which is carrying you to an uncertain destination. "You've got something," people will say, "but we don't know what it is." "We have to run more tests, but don't worry, it's probably not a serious problem." "You've got an undefined mass in your abdomen," people say, "but it could be nothing at all. Be easy on yourself. Try not to think about it."

Diagnosis is a patchwork of contradictions that forces you to admit that life is filled with imponderable uncertainties. How do we cope with these diagnostic uncertainties? Overcoming considerable doubt, some people attempt to march forward with confidence. "Nothing can happen to me, I'm fit," they might say. "I'm sure it will turn out okay." In some cases, the diagnostic experience, if my case is at all typical, has a numbing effect. If one becomes desensitized, she or he is protected from the distress that uncertainty precipitates. Another strategy is to push uncertainty into the background of consciousness. If you are consumed with work or family matters, you'll spend less time worrying about what's wrong. This strategy minimizes what social psychologists call "rumination"—thinking endlessly about a problem. Rumination promotes a wide assortment of negative emotional consequences. Most people, of course, combine bits and pieces of these strategies to cope with the diagnostic process.[10]

None of these strategies seemed to work well for me. I tried to convince myself that nothing was wrong. I told friends that I probably was okay, but the uncertainty of my situation prevented me from feeling positive about it. The endless series of sonograms, CAT scans, blood work, and biopsies made me numb, but the mental buffering that such insulation provides didn't protect me from uncertainty. The "painless" procedures I lived through filled me with fear; they also made me feel like a patient, a powerless subject. I tried throwing myself into my work. I taught with newfound energy. I made progress on a book manuscript. I volunteered to write book reviews and evaluate manuscripts. No amount of denial, numbness, or work, though, could erase my awareness of the "undefined mass" growing in my abdomen.

I longed to be more like the Songhay. Why couldn't I let fate carry me away to some unknown destination? Why couldn't I live with ambiguous uncertainty? The voice of Adamu Jenitongo came to me regularly in my dreams. He would say again and again: "Remember the path, remember the path." One night close to the end of the diagnosis ordeal, I recited *haro guso*, "the water container," an incantation that Sorko Djibo Mounmouni, the son of my first teacher, had taught me in 1977. It is designed to reinforce your power during difficult times.

HARO GUSU

I must speak to N'debbi, and my words must travel until they are heard. N'debbi was before human beings. He showed human beings the path. Now human beings are on the path. My path came from the ancestors [my teacher, my teacher's teacher]. Now my path is beyond theirs. The path is war. When there is war, men have thirty points of misfortune; women have forty points of misfortune. A person has many enemies on the path, enemies who will seek him out. The evil witches can search a person out with evil medicine, and a few of them will be overcome. They say that the evil genies will seek a person out and a few of them will be overcome. They say that the devil's children will seek a person out, and a few of them will be overcome, and the spirits of the cold will search a person out, and they, too, can be mastered. All of them are on the path; some of them can be mastered.

Chanted over a gourd filled with water, pulverized tree bark, powdered plants, and certain perfumes, this incantation, recited to the Songhay deity N'debbi, attracts back to its host body a soul that has been stolen by witches. Unlike most incantations among the Songhay, this one describes a path through life filled with potentially fatal conflicts that one must continually confront. Men have thirty points of misfortune; women, who rarely fare better than men in Songhay society, have forty points of misfortune.

If you are a Songhay person and expect to confront thirty or forty points of misfortune on your path, you spend much of your time trying to prevent an inevitable confrontation from completely devastating your life. Resisting the inevitability of misfortune is, as the Borg of *Star Trek* fame would say, futile. From this standpoint, the fiction of control dissipates.

Most Songhay people believe that points of misfortune are crossroads—spaces of danger in West African systems of thought. Although crossroads in Songhay country often conform to the familiar intersection model, many of them, especially in rural areas, are literally forks in the road. One path ends. Two new ones branch off, to the left and to the right. As you travel through life, you invariably come to crossroads, points of misfortune, spaces where the spirit and social worlds intersect, where forces in the spirit world "seek a person out." Standing upon a point of misfortune, you must decide which new path to follow. Here the wrong decision can have devastating consequences. If you make the wrong choice, you suffer through a shortened life filled with distress and illness. If you make the right choice, you live a longer life filled with laughter and health—until, of course, you have to negotiate the next point of misfortune. However you may view it, this reality is a hard one to bear.

Even so, it is a reality that makes sense for cancer patients. You have been told that you have cancer, an event that marks a point of misfortune. As you stand on that point of misfortune, you reconsider your life with what the French dramatist Antonin Artaud called "cruel" honesty. You have come to the end of one path—a fork in the road, which, you also realize, is a point of no return to the village of the healthy. Your life has been forever altered. You look back wistfully, but there is no way back to the past. Events have compelled you to decide which path to follow into the village of the sick. You also know that you alone will bear the consequences of that decision.

When I found myself standing on this point of misfortune in my oncologist's office and heard the news, I desperately wanted someone—anyone—to tell me what to do. Adamu Jenitongo's voice came to me, as it had many times in the past, but provided no direct guidance. When Songhay sorcerers confront a point of misfortune, as Adamu Jenitongo would say, they must find their own way. They must choose which path to take and bear the consequences. Confronting their own point of misfortune, cancer patients must make the same fateful choice.

That is the reality that the newly diagnosed cancer patient faces; it is a hard reality to bear.

CHAPTER TWO

Harmonizing the Bush at The Cancer Center

On a beautiful spring morning several weeks after I had been diagnosed with cancer, my brother Mitch took me to The Cancer Center for my first chemotherapy treatment. For over a month I had lived with the devastating knowledge that I had a tumor "the size of a small grapefruit," to quote Joel Rubin, my oncologist, growing in my abdomen. Because it was a slow-growing cancer, Joel hadn't felt it necessary to rush right into treatment. The biopsy of the bone marrow, moreover, had been clear of lymphoma cells. I therefore had one month between final diagnosis and first treatment to try to adjust to my new life as a cancer patient.

During that month I struggled to lead a "normal" life. I continued to teach. I traveled to New York City to talk to West African immigrants in Harlem and Chelsea, continuing my research project. I went to Chicago to testify as an expert witness in a political-asylum hearing. My friend Miriam dragged me to a couple of my favorite restaurants and to several films. I even made a weekend trip to the beach, where I own a small house.

Despite these distractions, nothing could keep me from thinking about what was happening to me. I worried constantly about my future. I spent hours reading about the side effects of chemotherapy, information that filled me with fear and anxiety. I geared myself up for body-wrenching nausea, bone-weary fatigue, and hair loss. I bought an electric razor to avoid excessive bleeding from a shaving cut—chemotherapy can reduce blood-clotting platelet levels—and a soft toothbrush to guard against painful mouth sores. I also read the literature about Rituxan, an antibody cloned from mice, which could be dripped into my bloodstream to kill lymphoma cells. Although this drug had fewer side effects than the chemotherapy medicines, it, too, could cause serious problems—fever, chills, and heart irregularities—especially the first time it was administered. I also didn't know if my medical insurance would cover its cost—more than five thousand dollars per dose.

I had suffered through hardships in the past. Professional struggles, family concerns, and most of all the ordeals I had faced as a young apprentice sorcerer had toughened me. But I wondered if I was tough enough for cancer. As much as possible, I made practical as well as emotional preparations for chemotherapy. But was I ready to face this physical and emotional trauma? Two days before my first treatment date, my brother Mitch had phoned to say that he wanted to accompany me. My appointment was scheduled for 11:45 A.M.

Mitch arrived on time, but for once did not exude his usual bright confidence and optimism. We drove to The Cancer Center in silence, avoiding the subjects of illness and life and death—something I had been thinking about for a month. For his part, Mitch might have been wondering if lymphoma had genetic links. During the previous year, our first cousin, my father's brother's son, had been diagnosed with lymphoma. Instead we made small talk, mostly about the best way to get from my apartment to The Cancer Center.

"We won't hit traffic that way, will we?" Mitch asked.

"I don't think so," I answered.

"How long does it take, usually?"

"About thirty-five minutes."

"And how many miles is it?"

"About fifteen."

We continued this scintillating dialogue for several miles of beautiful rolling hills. How strange it was that on such a traumatic day two men, for whom talk is so important, would have such an impoverished conversation. I earn a living by teaching and Mitch makes a living by talking people into contributing money for paralysis research.

Halfway to The Cancer Center I finally said it. "I'm scared."

Mitch put his hand on my arm. "I know. I'm scared, too. But I'm sure it will all turn out okay."

In this kind of situation what did "turn out okay" mean? Mitch hadn't read the literature on chemotherapy or on non-Hodgkin's lymphoma. Even though Joel Rubin had said that he expected me to live for decades, I wondered if I might nonetheless fall on the short side of the median survival line for all stages of NHL—seven to ten years.[1] I didn't want to talk about that possibility—neither did he—but it continued to lurk in the back of my mind. Silence became our friend as we crossed a narrow stone bridge that spanned a beautiful river. We snaked along a narrow country road, passing a horse farm equipped with a steeplechase course and spacious high-priced houses on postage-stamp lots. We finally inched our way into the small eastern Pennsylvania town where I taught and where I had decided to undergo cancer treatments.

At first glance The Cancer Center seems oddly out of place. Eastern Pennsylvania is filled with green rolling hills, horse farms, and majestic Quaker farmhouses, square and imposing, fashioned from locally quarried serpentine stone. In these small towns, like the one in which I work, houses are usually three-story turreted Victorian structures with porches; other homes are more Georgian in character—solid dark rectangular brick structures with walled gardens. In my university town, local authorities have attempted to maintain small-town quaintness.

Brick sidewalks have multiplied. Small specialty shops and up-scale restaurants have appeared. These additions project an image of an old-fashioned small town steeped in history. Like Georgetown in Washington, D.C., my hometown, which it re-sembles, the dark and closed spaces of this university town often generate a degree of reserve among its residents.

In stark contrast to its surroundings, The Cancer Center, like the county hospital across the street, is housed in a building that resembles a Spanish hacienda—bright, sunny cream-col-ored surfaces, open spaces, red tile roofs. The Cancer Center is located on the first floor of this building. Inside, the attempt to generate cheerful sunshine continues. There is a rectangular waiting room clothed in dappled cream-colored wallpaper. A beige Berber carpet mutes the glare of fluorescent lighting. Near the water fountain there is a photo of The Cancer Center's med-ical director. The photo had been part of a local magazine's fea-ture story about the "best" doctors in the Philadelphia area. This, too, has a soothing effect.

No degree of architectural planning or interior decorating, however, can alter the heavy reality of a room filled with cancer patients. Unlike my first zombie-like trip to The Cancer Center to receive the "official" diagnosis, on this visit my observational capacities were in full force. Conversation was muted. There was no laughter. A mother and her teenaged daughter, the color drained from their expressionless faces, sat stiffly and silently in their seats. A skeletal man, sporting perhaps a three-day growth of beard stubble, fidgeted in his chair. Parked next to him was a portable oxygen machine, marking him as a lung-cancer patient. A slender woman wearing a headscarf stared at the ceiling. One of her arms had swollen to the size one would expect in a woman three times her weight. I knew from my reading that removal of the lymph nodes can cause lymph-fluid backup, making limbs swell to elephantine proportions.

Mitch could not sit still. I knew that it must have been difficult for him to find himself in a room full of cancer patients. As a veteran of many diagnostic trials as well as a previous visit to The Cancer Center, I felt some distant kinship with these people. I still had my hair, and felt myself to be physically fit, and yet we all shared the burden of a grim diagnosis. Cancer always makes you confront death. This unwelcome and unexpected confrontation quickly erodes the gender, ethnic, and class differences that divide American society. At The Cancer Center, social differences among university professors, construction workers, and secretaries quickly fade away. Cancer makes us involuntary kin in the village of the sick. This realization sank me further into silence. Breaking the uncomfortable daydream, a woman called my name—a summons for me to give blood, a precondition for any chemotherapy treatment. I saw her waving to me from across the room, stood up, and walked over to her.

"Do you have your form?" she asked crisply as I approached the desk.

I handed her a sheet. The paper stipulated what kind of tests were to be performed, which in turn indicated how much of my blood she would draw. The blood room was bright, white and sterile. One section of it was occupied by machinery that computed the blood numbers. The rest of the room consisted of tables and four chairs with raised arms. I sat, lowered the chair's arm, and extended my left hand over the surface. The technician tied a latex tourniquet around my bicep. In search of a blood source, she tapped my veins. Finding a suitable candidate, she swabbed my arm with alcohol.

"You have beautiful veins. You must work out."

"That's right," I said, preparing myself for pain.

Her needle at the ready, she added: "This may sting a little bit."

I winced and looked away as she filled three vials with my blood. In short order, she extracted the needle and put a bandage over the incision site.

"You have a nice day," she said.

How could I have a nice day, I thought, when my body was about to be subjected to the long drip of chemotherapy drugs? Did the technician have any idea of the impact of what she had said? Probably not, I told myself, as I rolled down my sleeve and returned to the waiting room.

Just as I sat down, a young woman, dressed in street clothes rather than laboratory attire, walked into the waiting room. She had short blond hair and a pleasant smile. "Mr. Stoller," she said, looking my way. She carried a folder—my file.

Like a schoolchild, I raised my hand to verify my identity. She stepped closer to where I sat. "We need to weigh you and take your blood pressure before you see Dr. Rubin."

I followed her to a scale located in one corner of the waiting room.

"Should I take off my shoes?"

She smiled all-knowingly. "It doesn't matter."

I obediently stepped onto the scale, my heavy shoes anchoring to the platform.

She adjusted the various sliding controls until my "true" weight was indicated. She wrote down the number without comment. For once, I didn't care if I had gained weight. Still holding my file, she looked over to the blood-pressure machine. "Why don't you sit down and we'll take a reading?"

I wondered, continuing my silent critique of health care behaviors and procedures, why a clerk would be taking my blood pressure. When I went to my family physician, he took my blood pressure, which had been normal for as long as I could remember. Instead of questioning anything, I sat down and did what I was told. She wrapped a sleeve around my arm and pumped up the machine. The sleeve tightened around my arm like a tourniquet—much tighter than I had previously experienced.

"Nice weather we're having," she said personably.

"Very nice."

"The spring flowers are even beginning to bloom."

My attention, though, concentrated on a series of short beeps and then a long beep. The machine had recorded my blood pressure. The young woman had written it down, but didn't give me the reading.

"What was it?" I asked, trying to maintain my fast-fading composure.

"One-sixty over eighty," she said.

"That's high," I said. "Two weeks ago it was one-twenty over eighty."

"You know, people get nervous when they come here," she said.

"I guess so," I stated.

"Do you want to follow me back? The doctor will see you shortly."

"Thank you."

"Your friend can come back, too."

I turned to Mitch. "Do you want to come back?"

"Yes," he said quickly, trying to prepare for the next act of the play.

We followed the woman, passing the long L-shaped counter that separated the staff from the patients. Behind the staff space, I noticed a square room that held what seemed to be thousands of folders—medical records. We continued a short distance down the narrow hallway that formed a T-junction with a long corridor that ran the length of the building. We turned right. To the left we noticed doctors' offices; to the right we saw examination rooms. At the corridor's end, there was a corner conference room where nurses and doctors could go over test results, eat lunch, or have a staff meeting. Our guide opened the door to one of the examination rooms. "The doctor will be with you shortly," she said quickly.

We entered a typical medical-examination room—small, spare, square in shape, with two cushioned chairs and a swivel stool. We sat down and continued our silence. I began to shiver. Attempting to add a touch of warmth to the setting, someone had hung a painting—a house at the beach backgrounded by blue sky, puffy cumulus clouds, and soft surf.

This attempt to portray normality did not soothe me. Mitch continued to fidget. He asked me about Rituxan, the recently approved drug that might become part of my chemotherapy regime. Just as I began to recite the results of my research on the drug, Joel Rubin walked into this surreal setting. "Hello," he said with a smile.

Joel, who preferred first-name exchanges, sat down on the swivel stool and looked at my chart. I introduced him to my brother. They shook hands. "Mitch," I said proudly, "is the CEO of the Christopher Reeve Foundation."

They talked briefly about New Jersey, Mitch's home as well as the area where Joel had grown up. Joel wondered if the erratic stock market had made fund-raising more difficult. For me, this conversation seemed far away. I was thinking about side effects and my uncertain future.

"You'd be surprised," Mitch said. "Even in difficult times, people are willing to make major contributions for good causes."

"That's a good surprise," Joel said, as he opened my file. He swiveled toward me. "Your blood work is perfect," he said looking at the numbers. "I'll monitor your weight and pressure over the course of the treatments."

I sat silently in my chair. Mitch had the presence of mind to ask an important question. "How long will the treatments last?"

Joel shrugged. "That depends on how Paul responds. It could be as short as six months or as long as one year." He rolled the swivel chair closer to us and cleared his throat. "Have you thought about treatment options?" he asked.

On my previous visit to The Cancer Center, Joel had suggested three possible treatment alternatives for my non-

Hodgkin's lymphoma (NHL). The first was "watch and wait." NHL is a disease that can develop slowly. One may have lymphoma cells swelling lymph nodes or building bulky tumors, but not present any symptoms. One treatment alternative, as Joel explained, was to delay treatment until the onset of symptoms— weight loss, low-grade fevers, and night sweats.

Standard chemotherapy would be the second treatment alternative. I would receive three drugs, Cytoxan, vincristine, and prednisone. Nurses would administer the Cytoxan and vincristine through an intravenous drip. This process could last several hours. I would take 180 milligrams of prednisone a day, a massive amount, for seven days. At the end of three weeks, I'd come back for another treatment, and so on. I could expect at least eight cycles of chemotherapy. If at the end of eight cycles a CAT scan showed residual disease, I'd have to endure additional cycles of chemo. Joel had said that this treatment was usually effective for NHL patients like me.

The third treatment alternative would combine chemotherapy with Rituxan, the immunological medicine that contains antibodies that attach to specific antigens, molecules found on most lymphoma cells. The intercourse of antibody to antigen brings on the death of the malignant cell presumably without killing healthy cells—an advance over standard chemotherapy agents that destroy healthy as well as cancerous cells. Although it had been approved by the U.S. Food and Drug Administration for several years, Rituxan had been used only to treat lymphoma patients for whom chemotherapy had not worked or for previously treated patients whose cancer had returned. Very few people had received Rituxan as initial therapy. Fewer still had received it in tandem with chemotherapy.

"I've read the clinical studies," I began, struggling to sound professional, "and I'm impressed with Rituxan. The side effects are few and seem limited to the first infusion. It also seems very effective against the kind of NHL that I have." I paused. "What kind of impact do you think Rituxan will have on patients like me?"

Joel shrugged. "I don't know. There are a few clinical trials that suggest that Rituxan makes chemotherapy drugs more effective. But we really don't know."

Another of those troubling answers that fed my anxiety—a typical response to many of the treatment options offered to cancer patients. There have been so many new clinical developments—with only preliminary clinical results—in the treatment of lymphoma that physicians like Joel Rubin simply don't know the medical repercussions of every new therapy. In clinical trials, researchers use cancer patients—as volunteers—to test the effectiveness of new cancer drugs, but it takes years for specialists to obtain conclusive results. Despite the inconclusiveness of Joel's response, I appreciated his expression of uncertainty. "I'm also concerned about the cost," I added.

"It's very expensive," he said. "I've got several patients like you and their insurance has covered it. If yours doesn't, I can offer it to you at cost."

I looked at my brother. "I'd like to try Rituxan."

"Sounds like a good idea to me," Mitch said.

"If one of my family members had NHL," Joel added, "I'd recommend this combination therapy." He wrote down some notations on his chart, then excused himself in order to do some "calculations."

After he left, Mitch patted my arm. "You're doing the right thing, Paul," he said, his usual bright confidence returned.

Faced with an incurable disease, I decided I'd take risks that I might otherwise forgo. But I was still uncertain about my decision.

A few moments later Joel came back. "We are just about ready. This is how your treatment will work. First, you'll get some steroids to prevent nausea. Then you'll get a small dose of vincristine followed by Cytoxan. That will take about ninety minutes. We'll follow the Cytoxan with some Benadryl and Tagamet, which prepares you for Rituxan, which has to be given very slowly. The whole treatment process will take about five hours."

"That's a long time," Mitch observed.

At that moment the disruptive nature of my condition hit me like a Nigerien dust storm. Even if the chemotherapy treatments were successful, they would still change my life dramatically. Faced with these overwhelming circumstances, I struggled for strength. Slowly, I sensed a familiar tingling in my stomach—a sorcerous tingling. Blood surged through my veins. My senses finally began to wake up to the world in which I now found myself. I heard the soft voice of Adamu Jenitongo, my teacher and mentor: "You've found your way back to the path," he said. "Step onto it and walk forward."

Adamu Jenitongo had helped me once again. Because this moment was a crucial one in my life I now knew what to do—reconnect with what had given me strength in the past. I turned to Mitch. "Would you give me your hand?" I asked him.

I turned to Joel Rubin. "Could I hold your hand as well?"

He returned my gaze a bit skeptically.

"There are different paths to well-being," I explained softly. "You have your way of treating illness. I learned another perspective from my African teacher. I would like to rely on both now." I paused. "This treatment will bring physical and emotional disorder, pain, and suffering to my life. Disorder deepens illness. If I am going to get well I also need to follow the old ways of the sorcerers. I will try to harmonize the world in the way my teacher taught me. This will help me cope."

I took both of their hands and they patiently looked at me as I began to recite in Songhay an old incantation I had learned many years before.

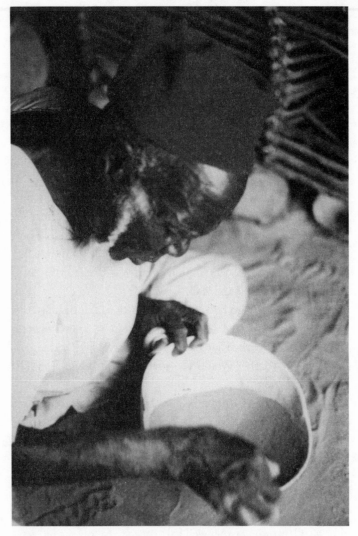

Adamu Jenitongo reciting the genji how *(1987). Photo: Paul Stoller*

In the name of the High God. In the name of the High God.
I speak to east. I speak to the west. I speak to the north. I speak
to the south. I speak to the seven heavens. I speak to the seven
hells. I am speaking to N'debbi and my words must travel until,

until, until they are known. N'debbi lived before human beings. He gave to human beings the path. He gave it to Soumana, and it was good for him. Soumana gave it to Niandou. Niandou gave it to Seyni. Seyni gave it to Jenitongo. Jenitongo gave it to Adamu and Adamu gave it to me. What was in their lips is in my lips. What was in their minds is in my mind. What was in their hearts is in my heart. Today I am infused with N'debbi and it is good for me. N'debbi has seven hatchets and seven picks. He gave the big rock, Wanzam, to Dongo. He gave power to the kings. He evades the capture of the blind. He evades the capture of the ancestors. The force— the force of heaven—protects all.

I finally loosened my grip and released their hands. Falling back in my chair, I took a deep breath. The words had comforted me. They made me feel more able to face what was ahead.

"What was that?" Joel asked.

"That is the *genji how*. It's an incantation that harmonizes the forces of the bush. The bush, here, is disharmonious. The words are in Songhay," I added. "It's the language of three million people in West Africa. I learned it when I lived there as a young man." Joel had known that I was an anthropologist. "I studied with a sorcerer for seventeen years. Like you," I told him, "I learned to be a healer—a different kind of healer. My teacher always said that there are many paths to well-being. I now understand more fully what he meant."

"I'd like to learn more about this," Joel stated.

I wondered what he thought about what had just happened. I truly appreciated his willingness to participate in a healing ritual that was so alien to his own training and background.

Shifting from the spiritual back to the practical, Joel stood up and retrieved my file. "Are you ready?" he asked.

I nodded.

"Follow me." We came to the end of the corridor and walked toward the front of the building to a nurse's station. Joel approached one of the oncology nurses, a tall and very attractive blond woman named Jennifer. If anyone were to drip poison into my body, I thought, let it be Jennifer.

Joel introduced us and handed Jennifer my file.

"It's good to meet you, Paul," she said with a smile. "I'll take very good care of you."

The *genji how*, I thought, must have already begun to work its magic! She stood up and led Mitch and me to the infusion room, a square space set off from the nurse's station by a wood counter; it was separated into four alcoves by dividers. Each treatment alcove held several medical recliners, flanked by upholstered chairs and swivel stools. Gold-plated art deco light fixtures attached to the cream-colored walls softened the effects of the fluorescent lighting. The linoleum tile looked cold and uninviting.

"Find yourself a seat," Jennifer said. "I'll go and mix your medicines."

She disappeared behind the nurse's station. I picked a chair closest to the nurses' station and the bathroom. Several patients, surrounded by family members and friends, were undergoing treatment. As chemotherapy medicines slowly dripped through plastic tubes and entered their bloodstream, they slept, talked quietly, read, or simply stared at the ceiling. My anxiety returned. I felt butterflies in my stomach. Perhaps I had been too quick to acknowledge the power of the *genji how*. Confronted by sobering circumstances, I again whispered the *genji how*, and followed that with an incantation for protection, which, like the *genji how*, I had learned many years before. The incantation is recited to Harakoy Dikko, goddess of the Niger River and mother-protector of human beings.

She gave birth to Suntunga. She gave birth to Muntanga. The Sah Tree. The Dugu Tree. The Wali Belin Tree. The Kasa Tobe Tree [sacred trees of Harakoy Dikko's domain under the Niger River]. The master of the small festival, Dikko; the master of the big festival, Dikko. The Koma kosi tree is in Zingi Komo, your village. Her hand comes to the sami tree; her hand returns to the sami tree. She nourishes the great river's bulanga tree.

Mother of peasants. Father of peasants. You must protect all the people in this room. You must bring into their mind-bodies the good feeling that brings on total peace and well being. May the words be true.

The words again brought me a degree of comfort. To complete the ritual, I spat very slightly on the linoleum floor. I hoped no one had noticed. Sorcerers spit after reciting an incantation so that their words carry to the east, the west, the north, and the south. Several minutes later, Jennifer returned.

æ æ æ

I had learned about the *genji how* many years before, while in Niger, at the end of a year of field research. Thinking of how much I had accomplished during the year filled me with a sense of pride. I had gathered enough ethnographic data to complete a dissertation on ritual language and local politics. More importantly, I had been quite unexpectedly initiated into Songhay sorcery. As part of this process, I had eaten *kusu*, the food of power that sorcerers occasionally consume. I had memorized incantations, learned to identify medicinal plants, and mixed sorcerous potions. I had even performed a sorcerous rite.

My apprenticeship had also enabled me to grasp the social impact of sorcery on the lives of people. A continuous stream of men and women of various ages brought their sufferings to Adamu Jenitongo, who diagnosed the source of the problem and offered a solution. Sometimes he prescribed a course of herbal medicines. Sometimes he suggested an animal sacrifice. On a few occasions he staged a spirit-possession ceremony to make offerings directly to the Songhay deities. In each and every case of affliction, sorcery appeared to be a means to the desired end, a restoration of health and well-being. Having had the privilege to "sit" with a man like Adamu Jenitongo, I saw myself as one of a small group of anthropologists who, through a combination of diligent fieldwork and happenstance, had been privileged to learn about sorcery from the inside.

My mentor did not share my self-congratulatory enthusiasm. Adamu Jenitongo knew nothing of anthropology or field methods. My youthful pride amused rather than impressed him. Sometimes I made him laugh so hard that he lost his balance. I would bring the wrong plant or mispronounce a Songhay word, or trip on a millet stump on my way to the bush to relieve myself—all cause for laughter. Over several months we had nevertheless developed a close relationship built upon what I hoped was a foundation of mutual respect.

Several days before I was to return to the United States to complete my graduate work, Adamu Jenitongo and I sat on a palm-frond mat in the shade of one of his conical straw huts. The midday heat blanched the sky. Dust hung like fog in the still air. In the distance a donkey brayed. The thumps of pestles in their mortars echoed in the dry air—lunch preparations.

An overflowing sleeveless black tunic and an ample pair of white drawstring trousers seemed to dwarf Adamu Jenitongo's spare body. A fez made of red felt topped his head. The tunic had two large side pockets, both of which bulged with his everyday necessities—kola nuts, which he savored regularly, loose tobacco, which he often kept nestled under his lip, a grater he used to shred the kola, which, because of his toothless condition, he couldn't chew. He would spend hours each day shredding kola, or sifting tobacco, both of which suppressed his appetite.

"Paul, you've learned a great deal," he said as he began to grate a kola nut.

"Thank you, *Baba*." I called him "father" out of respect for his age and wisdom.

He continued to grate. "And soon, you go back to America."

"Yes, in several days."

"May God protect you on your journey."

"May it be so," I said, following traditional Songhay conversational practices.

"Do you feel satisfied about what you have learned?"

"I do," I said with determination.

He shook his head and chuckled. "You do," he said, "and I don't."

"What do you mean?" I asked him, concerned and confused.

Rather than answering my question he took out a small leather pouch from one of his pockets, opened it, and spilled its contents—cowry shells—onto the mat. He put eleven shells in his hand and spoke to them for a brief moment. He then spit on them. Smoothing the sand near his position on the mat, he threw the shells. As he examined the configurations, he appeared to be listening to someone who wasn't there. He nodded to his invisible interlocutor. He chuckled and threw the shells again. He pointed to one shell that had piggybacked onto another. He shook his head, again listening to the invisible presence. "Yes, I see." He looked at me. "Do you see those shells?" he asked, referring to the piggybacked cowries.

I nodded.

"There is trouble on your path, my son."

I had had a good year. I was young. I felt safe and protected. Who would give me trouble, I wondered? "What kind of trouble?" I asked, a little less assured.

He threw the shells again. "I hear you," he said again to the presence I could neither see nor sense. "You have learned from me?" he asked me.

"That's right."

"You have eaten *kusu*?"

"Yes."

"Which means, my son, that you are on the path. When you are on the path you have many enemies. The path is war—even for someone like you. I see enemies on your path. They will test you. They will make you sick or tie you in knots."

"I see," I said skeptically.

"There will come times when you fear for your life. If that comes to pass, you must recite the *genji how*. It will help to protect you from your enemies."

"The *genji how?*" I asked, always the interested anthropologist.

Adamu Jenitongo spat some kola on the sand, gathered up his shells, and placed them carefully in the leather pouch. A rare cool breeze brushed against our faces. The smell of wood smoke mixed with frying onions wafted toward us. Slowly, he lifted his old body from the mat.

"Will you stay for lunch?"

I nodded eagerly. "But what about the *genji how?*" I asked, wondering if this was something else I had missed in my training.

"We'll talk later tonight."

That evening I left the house of a friend with whom I was staying and headed back toward Adamu Jenitongo's compound. A black moonless night made my flashlight-guided trip a slow and deliberate one. Vipers and puff adders came out at night and I wanted to be sure not to step on one of them. At midnight I could hear nothing except the whir of the wind and the crunch of my boots on cool dune sand. As I trudged up the dune behind the secondary school, I thought about what Adamu Jenitongo had told me. What had he seen in the shells? Although I had a great deal of respect for my Jewish heritage, I was not a particularly religious man. I wondered how a series of words would protect me from enemies. Despite my skepticism, it was an opportunity for me to learn an important incantation. Although I didn't think I'd ever have to use it for my own protection, I was eager to understand its power.

When I arrived at the entrance, an opening in the four-foot fence fashioned from millet stalks, I noticed a lantern glowing in one of the huts. Not wanting to awaken Adamu Jenitongo's family, I walked quietly to the hut and clapped softly to announce my arrival.

"Come in, my son," said a voice from inside.

Out of customary respect, I took off my shoes and socks, bent down, and pushed my way into the dimly lit hut. The lantern's flicker cast a parade of light and shadow over my mentor's jet-black face, which was as dry and taut as parchment. Although deep lines furrowed his forehead, the rest of his face was remarkably free of wrinkles. His eyes, even in the dim light, shone like beacons. Such eyes, which sometimes displayed a soft kindness, could pierce through a person's facades and seize her or his essence. I now realize that when our eyes locked during our first encounter, he had quickly figured me out. Taking in his magnificent face, I sat down opposite him.

He spoke in a whisper. "The *genji how* is very powerful; it balances the forces of the bush. Use it before you engage in sorcery or whenever you feel threatened."

Quite moved by what was about to transpire, I nodded.

"These words come from my ancestors. They are sacred. They are stronger than you and me. You must respect them. You must take care for them. You must never forget them." He paused for a moment. "Do you hear what I'm saying?"

"Yes, I do, *Baba*." In truth, I barely understood the emotional and philosophical importance of what he said. Being impatient, I wanted to get on with it.

"Then you are ready to receive the words."

With that, he patiently taught me the incantation, the words of which were understood to travel to the four cardinal directions as well as to the seven heavens and seven hells. After several hours, during which I forgot or mispronounced words, Adamu Jenitongo seemed satisfied with my progress. It had been a long night, but excitement filled me with energy.

"I know that the *genji how* is now in your heart," he said, "and will remain there. Recite it one more time for me."

I did as I was told.

In the name of the High God. In the name of the High God.
I speak to east. I speak to the west. I speak to the north. I speak
to the south. I speak to the seven heavens. I speak to the seven
hells. I am speaking to N'debbi and my words must travel until, until, until they are known. N'debbi lived before human
beings. He gave to human beings the path. He gave it to
Soumana, and it was good for him. Soumana gave it to Niandou. Niandou gave it to Seyni. Seyni gave it to Jenitongo. Jenitongo gave it to Adamu and Adamu gave it to me. What was
in their lips is in my lips. What was in their minds, is in my
mind. What was in their hearts is in my heart. Today I am infused with N'debbi and it is good for me. N'debbi has seven
hatchets and seven picks. He gave the big rock, Wanzam, to
Dongo. He gave power to the kings. He evades the capture of
the blind. He evades the capture of the ancestors. The force—
the force of heaven—protects all.

After he nodded his approval, I asked the aged sorcerer
about the meaning of the incantation. Some of the elements
were clear. I knew about N'debbi, the intermediary between the
High God and human beings. I knew about the seven heavens
and seven hells, a concept grafted from Muslim theology. I knew
about Wanzam, the rock that harbored the power of Dongo, the
feared deity of thunder. I understood the deep genealogy that
the incantation entailed. N'debbi's force, moreover, came from
his control of the Word. He gave the Word and took it back,
which meant that he taught human beings powerful incantations and received these same words when human beings re-
quested the power of his services. Although I knew that he was
tired, I had to ask Adamu Jenitongo one last question.

"How can these words protect me?"

The old man chuckled and he nodded his head. "I cannot tell
you that. You must seek your own answers."

I began to protest this unsatisfactory response.

"Each person on the path," he interjected, "must find his

own way, his own answers." He yawned again. "One day you will understand." He lay down on his mat. "Sleep here, if you like." "No, no, *Baba*. Thank you, but I'll go back."

Several days later I left Tillaberi and returned to America. After much reflection, I concluded that the *genji how* was a beautiful poem that I had committed to memory. When I transcribed and translated it, the *genji how* became an important piece of anthropological data that revealed some key themes in Songhay culture. I didn't believe at that time that a sequence of words, however poetic, could harmonize the forces of the bush or protect me from voracious sorcerers.

⌘ ⌘ ⌘

The intellectual legacy of Western philosophy shaped, in large measure, my initial skepticism of the *genji how*'s power. Although recent debates among scholars have questioned the legitimacy of the scientific worldview, anthropology has remained very much a social science. In the 1970s my disciplinary mentors taught me that social scientists must develop and maintain a critical vantage from which they doubt the received truths of the past and are critical of the reigning theories of the present. Truth, I learned, is an unstable condition. To paraphrase William James, truth is like a check. It's good only as long as there is money in the bank.

Skepticism, of course, has been central to the Western pursuit of knowledge. Its roots stretch well into classical Greek philosophy. In the third century A.D. Sextus Empiricus underscored the philosophical need to doubt everything. Echoing Sextus, in the eighteenth century David Hume expressed the belief that reason itself was laced with contradictions. For Hume no truth or sense impression was final, except perhaps the spirit of inquiry.[2] In its more modern application, skepticism has two orientations: epistemic, doubts about taken-for-granted beliefs, and ontological, doubts about claims of existence.

In anthropology, these concerns are especially important in the study of the religious practices of non-Western peoples. Many Songhay, for example, claim that spirits exist and take the bodies of mediums and that magical words can heal, maim, or kill a person. True to my training, I believed that my task was to uncover a rational explanation for such "apparently irrational beliefs."[3]

Physicians, of course, hold similar beliefs about rationality and science. They tend to be skeptical of alternative medicine or nonscientific approaches to healing the body.[4] It makes them cautious about diagnosis, a practice, as we have seen, that is laced with uncertainty and doubt. It makes them hesitant to endorse such practices as reflexology, herbalism, or Reiki, which are used by an increasingly large population of people, including, of course, people facing an incurable disease. Perhaps the degree of a person's skepticism about illness, cures, or "apparently irrational beliefs" devolves from her or his standpoint in the world. From within the village of the healthy, skepticism makes good sense; it has advanced our knowledge of and control over the world by leaps and bounds. From within the village of the sick, in which death is your constant companion, skepticism fades away with other commonplace beliefs that people maintain in the village of the healthy. In the village of the sick, you begin to wonder if skepticism is good for your body.

❀ ❀ ❀

On my first trip to Wanzerbé, the feared village of Songhay sorcerers, I thought that skepticism enabled the anthropologist to produce authoritative knowledge. Having never been very sick, the idea that skepticism might be good or bad for my body had never crossed my mind. During that trip, after all, I hadn't needed an incantation to protect me from supernatural forces. As Wanzerbé is the most feared center of sorcery in Niger, no traveler would go there without a local escort. Despite its reputation, I found Wanzerbé to be a pleasant village filled with kind and gracious people.

When I first went there early in 1977, I had not yet eaten *kusu*, which marks the formal beginning of the sorcerer's education, nor yet received the *genji how*, which, as I later learned, is the central resource in a sorcerer's defense. I had learned a little about sorcery and was curious about the history and people of Wanzerbé. Luckily, my housemate, Idrissa, was from Wanzerbé and wanted to visit his family. He suggested that I accompany him home.

Getting from Mehanna on the Niger River to Wanzerbé, 120 kilometers to the northwest, near the Niger–Burkina Faso border, would prove to be difficult. Idrissa suggested that we take bush taxis—usually a small Peugeot truck with a canvas-covered carrier lined with benches bolted to the floor. Taxis would come to Mehanna market and take us to Tera, the regional administrative center. From there, we could get a ride to Wanzerbé. I preferred the less efficient and more direct mode of transportation—horseback. I had a horse, a substantial Arabian stallion, and I offered to rent one for Idrissa. In this way, I could see more villages, get a feel for the desolate countryside, and meet new people. Idrissa agreed, but wondered if I, a Westerner, was up a 240-kilometer round trip in the considerable heat of March.

We left early one morning, a cool Niger River breeze at our backs. We followed a road over the massive dunes that eventually gave way to a red clay plain strewn with rocks. We saw no other living thing and heard only the rhythmic clack of horse hooves on hard clay. The hot desert wind, the harmattan, blew relentlessly in our faces. After about two hours, we came upon another range of dunes and saw Lugi, a village of one hundred people who lived mostly in straw huts. Idrissa had a friend who lived there in a two-room mud-brick house. With customary Songhay hospitality, Idrissa's friend welcomed us, had his son water our horses, and served us tea. It was good to get off the horses, get out of the wind, and take some refreshment. This respite, though, was a brief one, for Idrissa was determined that we get to Bankilare, our first day's destination, before sunset. All too quickly, we finished our tea, mounted our horses, and rode toward a range of dunes to the northwest. I imagined myself deep in the Sahara, isolated from civilization. These thoughts reduced the discomfort of heat, wind, and horse gait. Later in the day we came upon a small encampment of Fulani nomads who offered us milk as we rested in the shade of a tamarind tree. We were also able to fill our almost empty canteens.

We resumed our trip and soon found ourselves in a vast track of treeless plain. The afternoon sun burned our faces. My body ached. Toward dusk, we finally rode into the outskirts of Bankilare, a small town inhabited by Tuareg—the famous blue men of the desert. Idrissa led us to a relative's compound. His cousin Altinne served on the border patrol. Each day, he'd mount his camel to patrol the Niger-Mali border, which was twenty kilometers to the north. He received us warmly. His wife served us tea. That evening we shared the family meal of rice and mutton. I felt proud of myself for having traveled so far in difficult circumstances. Idrissa told his cousin that I was courageous—for a white man, of course. That night, under a star-filled sky, I slept like a baby, on an army cot.

In the morning we sipped Nescafé and drank gourds of millet gruel, thanked our host, and departed for Wanzerbé. The dunes gave way to vast clay plains offset by brown jagged mountains. At midday we reached a village where Idrissa's aunt prepared us a lunch of freshly slaughtered chicken over rice smothered with sesame sauce. We ate, thanked our hostess, watered our horses, and prepared for the last leg of our trip.

"In two hours," Idrissa said. "We should be in Wanzerbé."

After what seemed a relatively short ride along a trail that meandered through sandstone buttes, we came to Surgumey, the mountain that overlooked Wanzerbé and the site of a yearly sacrifice that was believed to protect Wanzerbé residents from illness and bad fortune. From our vantage near the summit of Surgumey, we saw the village below us. Its two neighborhoods sat atop dunes that bordered a tributary of the Niger River, the Garuol.

"That's Wanzerbé," Idrissa stated with pride.

As we entered the village, children surrounded us. They greeted Idrissa and me and sang praise-songs. As soon as we dismounted, scores of Idrissa's beaming relatives came to greet him. They welcomed me as a guest. We stayed for several days. Each night, Idrissa's family served us rice, millet, and tea. One relative even killed a sheep in our honor.

No one talked about Wanzerbé's considerable reputation as the feared village of sorcerers and witches. We were honored guests—objects of gracious hospitality. I wondered if the fabled status of the village of sorcerers had been exaggerated. Wanzerbé seemed like a typical Songhay village. After one festive week, we returned to Mehanna without incident.

Two years later I went back to Wanzerbé to deepen my knowledge of Songhay sorcery. Circumstances there had changed considerably. The harvest had been a poor one. People had had little to eat and less to share with guests. No one could afford to kill a sheep to honor visitors. My status had also changed. I was no longer a white man who had ridden a horse from Mehanna to Wanzerbé. Having studied the ways of sorcery under the guidance of Adamu Jenitongo, I now posed a potential threat to the Wanzerbé sorcerers who, having not known of my interest in their secrets, had been discreet during my first visit. They now knew that I was Adamu Jenitongo's apprentice. This fact meant that my journey to the fabled village of sorcerers would become a test of my sorcerous capacities. Among Songhay sorcerers, knowledge is power, especially when it can be used to heal, maim, or kill. Like most specialists who possess powerful knowledge (and here one thinks especially of physicians) the sorcerers of Wanzerbé wanted to limit its distribution.

Was I worthy of acquiring such knowledge? I had thought that Adamu Jenitongo had sent me to Wanzerbé to seek new sorcerous knowledge. But Wanzerbé sorcerers had no interest in teaching me their secrets. Instead, as Adamu Jenitongo had known, they would want to determine how much I had learned. I recited the *genji how* to protect myself, I had passed the "tests," and had even managed to overcome temporary paralysis. That experience also introduced me more fully to the rigors and dangers of the Songhay world of sorcery, a world in which one misstep could well result in illness or death. I had learned more respect for the ways of sorcery. The *genji how* had become more than a mere poem for me. Its words bore consequence. I believed that on my last visit to Wanzerbé they had saved my life. Despite this success, sorcery had frightened me. I left Wanzerbé and resolved to never return.

What was it in this windswept village that had the power to heal, but also to maim and kill? Did I really want to explore more fully this mysterious world so radically different from my own? As a social scientist I tried to understand the beliefs and ways of others. I attempted to discover rational explanations for what, on the surface, seemed like a set of bizarre understandings and strange behaviors. More personally, I had great respect for whatever brought others solace in difficult circumstances. In many respects, sorcery fit this criterion. But as I learned in Wanzerbé, the ways of sorcery could also be brutal. After much reflection, I displaced some of my skepticism and suspended my disbelief. I decided to continue the study of sorcery to more fully understand the ways of Songhay culture. By electing to continue on sorcery's path, I would maintain my master-apprentice relationship with Adamu Jenitongo, whom I had grown to love as a father.

When I returned to my "Western" life, I tried to maintain a tie to the ways of sorcery. This link comforted me and reaffirmed my connection to Adamu Jenitongo. I made a small altar in my home. It is a low round table covered with a black tunic that represents Dongo, deity of thunder. Positioned at the center of the table surface is a *batta,* a sacrificial container. My *batta* is a simple glass jar that Adamu Jenitongo gave to me in Niger. The jar, the lid of which reads "Lasco Spiced Cut Herring," is entwined with black thread—also representing Dongo. Inside the jar is the stuff of sacrifice—aromatic twigs and roots, the residue of years of blood and perfume offerings, and an assortment of rings that "sit" and "drink." Surrounding the jar is an array of small perfume jars arranged in an arc that follows the curve of the table. These are also associated with the spirits of the Songhay pantheon. Between the *batta* and the table's back edge lay two small satchels, one white, one black. The white satchel contains divining shells; the black one holds smaller satchels of pulverized tree barks. Just behind the table a small hatchet covered in red leather rests on two nails hammered into the wall. A small bell attached to its head marks it as Dongo's hatchet. Every Thursday and Sunday, days of the Songhay spirits, I make offerings. I first recite the *genji how* to set the world straight, for offerings cannot be made in disharmonious circumstances. Then I sing Dongo's praise-song and feed the hatchet with his favorite perfume. This offering showers one's path with grit and determination. After reciting the *genji how* on Sundays, I sing the praise-song for Harakoy Dikko, goddess of the Niger River. This offering provides protection along the path.

I also recite the *genji how* when I do "work" for friends and family, an attempt to use what I've learned to bring them increased health, harmony, and well being. On rare occasions when I throw divining shells, I'd first recite the *genji how*—again, to set the world in order. Shells are read on Thursdays and Sundays, for it is only on days of the spirits that shells "speak" to the diviner. If the world is chaotic, the shells keep their silence—even on Thursdays and Sundays. If I agreed to cleanse a house of disharmony caused by argument, ill will, or death, I'd also recite the *genji how.*

Several years ago when the husband of a friend died sud-

denly, I volunteered to go to her house to cleanse it. Carrying a
bowl of milk, I went from room to room. In every room, I walked
to the corners, recited the *genji how*, and then sprayed milk.
These measures seemed to lift the spirits of my friends and family and gave them an increased sense of vitality. This "success" reinforced the spiritual connection that Adamu Jenitongo had
established between us.

❀ ❀ ❀

Even though I had practiced sorcery for many years, it was not
until I became a cancer patient that the rituals of Songhay sorcery took on deeper meanings. As a young apprentice sorcerer
I had considered these rituals a weapon in my sorcerous arsenal.
I believed then that sorcery was much like gunfighting in Hol-
lywood westerns. Gunfighters practiced and dueled to become
"the fastest gun in the West," which meant that their very presence injected fear—and respect—into any atmosphere. Gunfighters, like sorcerers, felt no sense of morality. They felt little
or no remorse about the people they wounded or killed on their
way to the top. Being top gun, though, seemed a mixed blessing.
Out of fear, people paid them considerable deference. By the
same token, a skillful challenger could at any moment propose a
gunfight, which could result in the top gun's death. In worlds of
sorcery, there are "top guns" who are being continuously challenged—often with mortal consequences. Despite the power of
my weapons (potions, power objects, and the *genji how*), I didn't
possess the proper belief and stamina to harness sorcerous
power.

I therefore used the *genji how* to perform small tasks—offerings, divination, ritual purifications. I recited the *genji how* the
way most people recite prayers—without thinking deeply about
its meaning. I recited it to set the world straight for moments of
time as well as, after Adamu Jenitongo's death, to honor the

memory of my late mentor. The *genji how* had again become a sequence of words.

And yet, when I sat in Joel Rubin's examination room the words of the *genji how* surged like a current into my consciousness. They had become central weapons in my fight against lymphoma. I finally realized that I had misunderstood the deep meaning of the incantation. It was a sorcerous weapon that could divert death. It was a sequence of words that could reestablish harmony in chaotic circumstances. What I hadn't realized was that the power of the incantation—not to forget the wisdom of Songhay sorcery—comes from the combination of two components: disharmony and peace. By creating harmonious peace in the infusion room, the *genji how* primed me to confront the devastation of cancer.

❊ ❊ ❊

Twenty-five years after Adamu Jenitongo first introduced me to the world of sorcery, I revisited that strange universe. My knowledge of sorcery provided me with comfort. My own religious background, Judaism, gave me a set of abstract principles about the world in which I lived, but provided no concrete formulas for dealing with an unexpected and incurable disease. Sorcery, by contrast, provided a reassuring set of principles about how to live in the world. And yet, how many cancer patients, as one of my friends put it, have "sorcery in their pocket"? Before I became a cancer patient, I would have said that very few people could make use of such a tool. I would have also said that to have access to sorcery is a mixed blessing. Although it can make you strong, it also makes you vulnerable.

Time and experience have taught me that everyone, especially cancer patients, can benefit from the world of sorcery. As I now understand it, sorcery is more than a set of esoteric practices; it is a way carrying oneself in the world. The *genji how,* for example, is an intrinsic part of sorcerous ritual. Its powerful words prepare a setting for sorcerous actions. Sorcerers, as already mentioned, always begin their work with ritual texts like the *genji how*. Sometimes they use such texts to divert death or sickness. Above and beyond its specific uses, the *genji how* is a ritual incantation, something that is said the same way and in the same context day in and day out, year in and year out. Through the recitation of the *genji how* the sorcerer attempts to maintain a semblance of order in the world.

Like the *genji how*, rituals set the world straight. Anthropologists usually associate rituals with religious life and suggest that they constitute that which is considered sacred. Religious services, for example, are a collection of ritual incantations (prayers, hymns, and invocations) that bring to worshippers a sense of calm and peace. In search of calm and peace, people seek solace in churches, synagogues, and mosques—especially when they must confront trying personal experiences or troubling public events.

Rituals, however, also work their magic in the routine world of everyday life. Each of us has her or his personal rituals. Doing certain things when we wake up or go to sleep may help to set the world straight and bring us a sense of calm. Some people may run or stretch every morning before going to work; other people may take a soothing bath at night before going to bed. I like to wake early, brew coffee, and write. When we are able to perform these personal rituals, they give us a good feeling. They make us feel, if only for a little while, that we can generate and maintain a measure of control over our lives.

When you learn that you have cancer, the world spins out of control. You are thrown into a world of medical procedures and inconclusive diagnoses. What's more, you have to interact with technicians and medical professionals, many of whom can be insensitive. The texture of your social relationships changes. Your friends and family may shower you with too much attention and concern; they may talk too much about your disease. Some of your friends and family may seek comfort in denial; they avoid the subjects of illness and death. Meanwhile, you find yourself in the vortex of a whirlwind. No matter what kind of support you have from friends, family, and professionals—and the importance of this support cannot be overestimated—the cancer cells have appeared in your body, which means that ultimately you, like the African sorcerer, must face your fate alone.

Confronting cancer is a frighteningly lonely proposition. How do you deal with your isolation? How do you face your fate? Songhay sorcerers have one suggestion; they say that you should diligently perform personal rituals. Throughout my treatments for lymphoma, I tried to follow this principle. Seated in the recliner in the infusion room of The Cancer Center, I'd recite the *genji how* and follow it with an incantation for protection. Once I had spit lightly into the air so that my words would infuse the infusion room with old and powerful sounds, I'd spread a piece of Malian *bogolanfini* fabric—black geometric patterns on brown homespun cloth—over the drab brown table next to my chair. I would take my jazz tapes—Coltrane, Gillespie, Mingus, and Hamilton—and put them on the cloth next to my Walkman and several Ironman energy bars. When my oncology nurse came in to connect me to the intravenous line, I would put on my earphones and fly away to some distant spot in John Coltrane's musical universe. Throughout my treatments, I never varied my ritualistic routine: *genji how,* incantation for protection, cloth, jazz, and Ironman bars. The routine helped me to endure the five-to-six-hour treatment sessions. In my social and physical isolation, they helped me to confront the physical and emotional pain that I was experiencing. They gave me a degree of control over an uncontrollable situation. I am also convinced that they primed the immune system to purge my body of lymphoma cells. After three treatments, the combination of chemotherapy and Rituxan had shrunk my abdominal tumor by 50 percent. What's more, I hadn't lost my hair, and had retained enough energy to teach, write, and even travel a bit.

Engaging in personal rituals, of course, cannot guarantee a successful course of chemotherapy, but it *can* assure, I think, a certain sense of personal control, which goes a long way toward maintaining quality of life. Any cancer patient can engage in this kind of ritual. Before treatment, you might recite a certain prayer or poem, like the *genji how*, that gives you comfort. You might wear clothing that makes you feel confident. You might bring food that fuels your energy. You might bring music that sends you on a soothing dreamlike journey. These personal rituals transform a clinical encounter into a meaningful personal odyssey. They bring you peace, following the wisdom of the *genji how*, so that you can be ready for what life presents on your path.

❀ ❀ ❀

When I lived in Niger I learned that rituals can also prepare a person to see things more clearly—an important lesson for the apprentice sorcerer or a person who has to confront a serious illness like cancer. Early on in my apprenticeship, Djibo Mounmouni, the son of my first teacher, asked me to assist him in a sorcerous rite. His client, a prosperous shop owner, had been ill for weeks. He had a bad cough, night sweats, and had lost weight. The shop owner had consulted the nurse at the local dispensary, who gave him antibiotics, which had no effect on his condition. He then went to the regional hospital. Nurses took samples of his blood, but found nothing abnormal. He went to the national hospital in Niamey. Doctors at the hospital put him through a battery of tests, none of which were conclusive. Believing that the shop owner's illness was in his head, the doctors suggested that he return home. After his return to Mehanna, the condition further deteriorated. Giving in to the twists and turns

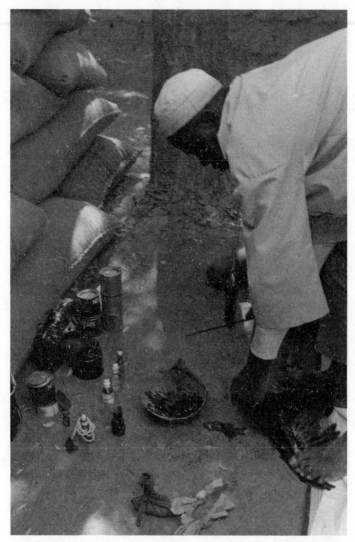

Sorko Djibo Mounmouni making an offering to the spirits. Photo: Paul Stoller

of fate, he prepared for death. As a last resort, he asked Djibo
Mounmouni to intervene.

I accompanied Djibo on this mission, eager to see how sorcery might help someone suffering from a serious illness. We

walked into the man's spacious compound. The sick man had built three cement houses that were surrounded by towering acacia and eucalyptus trees. We found him lying on a stick bed in the shade of the trees. He turned from side to side and talked to himself. Sweat had beaded on his forehead. Djibo felt his cheek.

"He's got a high fever," he observed. "It must be witchcraft." He then stated resolutely, "I know what to do."

He found a large white porcelain basin and filled it with water. "Come closer, Paul, so you can see and learn," he ordered. He took from his pocket a small vial of perfume and emptied it into the basin. He then took several satchels from his pocket. From them, he spread an assortment of powders—dried tree barks and grasses—on the water's surface. He recited an incantation that established a genealogy of power, naming the sorcerers of the past who had possessed it and passed it down from generation to generation. The incantation went on to describe the points of misfortune on the path of life. It mentions all the enemies one can confront and how the sorcerer can vanquish them. When Djibo finished his recitation, he spat into the ablution so that the power of old words entered into the water.

Djibo then asked the shop owner's wife to wash her husband with the fragrant ablution.

His work completed, we left the compound. I asked Djibo if we were, indeed, finished and if the man was cured.

Djibo laughed. "Of course not. A witch has stolen the man's soul. We have to find it and free it. Then the strong fragrance of the ablution will attract the man's soul back to his body and he will be healed."

I remained skeptical. I knew that according to the Songhay a person consists of flesh, the soul, and the life force. The life force resides in the heart. It is given at birth and leaves the heart at death. Flesh is flesh. The soul is a person's shadow—a person's immaterial being. As long as a person's soul and body remain united, she or he remains healthy. When witches steal the soul, they hide it in various places. When that occurs, victims suffer from debilitating illnesses—fevers, body aches, loss of appetite, insomnia. If witches consume the victim's soul, he or she dies. I wondered how a witch, even if he or she existed, could eat a soul?

Djibo harbored no such doubts. "Follow me," he ordered. "We're going to find the shopkeeper's soul." We trudged up the sandy road until we reached the outskirts of town. The mud-brick compounds of longtime residents gradually gave way to the grass huts and millet-stalk fences of new arrivals. Beyond the newest neighborhoods, we noticed several piles of millet husks that formed mounds on the sand.

Saying nothing, Djibo walked toward the mounds and got down on his hands and knees. He sifted through the husks. "Praise be to God," he proclaimed. "Praise be to God."

I watched him as he worked.

Djibo finally stood up and shook his head. "I liberated the soul of the shopkeeper." Noticing the puzzled expression on my face, he pointed his finger at me. "You look, but you don't see. You listen, but you don't hear. You touch, but you don't feel." He shook his head. "You have much to learn." He paused a moment. "It will take years for you to see, hear, and feel the world."

❀ ❀ ❀

Djibo's comments bothered me. He had talked about images, sounds, and textures that did not exist in the "real" world—at least the world as I knew it. How could I see something that was invisible? How could I hear something that made no sound? How could I feel something that had no tangible surface? It did indeed take me many years to understand that Djibo's comments encapsulated the central tenets of Songhay sorcery. It takes a lifetime to learn how to "see," "hear," and "feel" the world.

Among the first steps of my education in sorcery was learning how to see. For sorcerers, to see is to look deeply into the past, present, and future—the art of divination. Songhay sorcerers use one of two methods to see—geomancy and divining shells. The geomancer traces lines in the sand and uses a complex numerology to read past, present, and future. Although this technique is rarely used in Niger, variations of the practice are widely employed throughout West and Central Africa.

Divining shells are more commonly used in Niger. Before Adamu Jenitongo taught me how to see, I observed scores of divining sessions. The sorcerer typically throws small white shells—the cowry shells that had once been used as currency in precolonial Niger—to assess a person's situation or to discover the source of his or her misfortune or illness. After the sorcerer has read the shell configurations, he or she prescribes a course of action—a series of animal sacrifices, an offering to the blind, or a course of herbal medicines. Anthropologists have written extensively about divination. For the most part they see it as a complex mathematical system that uses sophisticated scales of probability to deliver results.[5] I relied on this anthropological literature to try to make sense of the divination sessions I had witnessed. Despite the insights that this information provided, I still failed to grasp the relationship between the shell patterns and the sorcerer's observations. I did learn that if the small opening of the shell faces up, it is "female." Conversely, if the large opening faces up, the shell is "male." Beyond this primary distinction, I could make little sense of how the infinite combinations of male and female indicated betrayal, jealousy, illness, or death.

After a session with Adamu Jenitongo, I asked my mentor about how he read shells.

"That," he said, "I cannot tell you. You must learn for yourself. You must receive 'sight' from Wambata."

Wambata was the headstrong Songhay spirit that lived near

cemeteries. As a young female spirit, she dwelled in the sky with her brothers and sisters. For many years they tolerated her willfulness. But toleration, according to the legend of Wambata, had its limits—even for spirits. One day her siblings threw her out of the sky. The fall from grace broke both of her legs. Wounded, she crawled to a cemetery, where she married the genie of death. Their spirit children became the Songhay spirits of death—the spirits of the cold. "What does Wambata have to do with seeing?" I asked.

"I will try to give you sight," Adamu Jenitongo said, "and then you can better understand Wambata."

He invited me into the conical spirit hut and asked me to sit down on a palm-frond mat. He took out three large red kola nuts that had been stored in water in a small clay pot for three days.

"Put these over your eyes," he ordered.

He then began to recite a series of incantations. Sitting there with the cool kola nuts pressed against my closed eyes, I wondered how this ritual might give me sight. Listening to these incantations impelled me to think about what Adamu Jenitongo had already taught me about the Songhay view of divination. The world, according to Songhay belief, is a dangerous place filled with potential misfortune. You expect to confront all sorts of trouble—betrayal, loss, and illness—along your path. Although you cannot expect to evade misfortune, which is the norm rather than the exception in life, you can try to be prepared for it. One way to do so is divination. A diviner can throw shells to pinpoint where you will confront misfortune on life's path, and what type of misfortune it will be. Forewarned in this manner, you might be able to take preemptive measures—offerings, a course of fortifying medicines—to better confront the trouble that fate invariably brings your way.

This viewpoint did not seem terribly exotic to me. It made me think of my grandmother's considerable fear of the evil eye. Like many Songhay people, she saw misfortune in every nook and cranny of the world. Thinking that the evil eye would punish self-assurance, ostentation, and beauty, she, like many other eastern European Jews, Greeks, and Italians stressed modest self-presentation and avoided making positive statements. You could say something positive in my grandmother's household, but only if you followed the statement by saying, "May God protect me from the evil eye." In my grandmother's world there were no people like Adamu Jenitongo, someone who could see trouble long before it appeared.

Hearing the praise-names of Wambata, spirit of death and goddess of divination, jolted me from my reveries. Adamu Jenitongo recited her praise-poem with emphasis and deliberation. It is a poem that describes the clairvoyant powers of a willful female spirit, the mother of death.

WAMBATA

> She is the essence of cold. She is big and she is strong. She is stronger than any woman. She is stronger than any man. She sees all and knows all. She looks into the sun and sees. She looks into the moon and sees. In the obscurity of fresh milk she sees clarity. In the obscurity of blood, she sees clarity. She comes to the place of death. Whether she is in front of or behind you, she wreaks havoc. Praise to the mother of Ma Suu, of Ma Susu, of Genji Ceri, of Bong'izey, of Na Wao, and of Towey [all spirits of the cold; i.e, death].

I understood clearly Wambata's capacity to see clarity—the past, present, and future—in the brightness of the sun, in the glow of the moon, in a bowl of milk, or in a pool of blood. I wondered, though, how Wambata's capacities might be extended to me.

"You now have vision," Adamu Jenitongo stated when he had finished.

"You mean that if I throw shells I'll see the past, present, and future?"

The old man chuckled. "Why do you want to do things so quickly? I have given you the potential for vision. You must find your own way to sight. Be patient. Your path will open in front of you." He paused a moment. "Maybe your path will open next year," he said. "Maybe five years or even ten years from now. Your path might never open, my son." He paused to put some grated kola under his lip. "It depends upon you and Wambata." He pulled a leather pouch from one of the pockets in his tunic. He counted thirteen cowry shells and put them into a cloth satchel, which he tied shut. "Take these. They will help you to see."

I thanked him and took the shells and put them into the pocket of my tunic.

"Be careful with the shells. They have been sacrificed upon and then buried in a termite hill for seven years. These are Wambata's shells. She will not speak through other shells."

Late that afternoon I returned to a friend's house and eagerly attempted to throw the shells to divine his future. The configurations did not reveal anything about my friend's past, present, or future. I did not hear Wambata's voice. I doubted that Wambata could show me the way to clairvoyance.

One year later I returned to Niger to continue my studies with Adamu Jenitongo in Tillaberi. He taught me sorcerous incantations and allowed me to observe sorcerous rites, but had nothing to say about divination. After several weeks at his compound, I asked him to again teach me about the cowry shells.

"Maybe it's time for you to visit your friends in Mehanna."

I followed his advice, not knowing how my friends in Mehanna, the town where I conducted my early field research, could help me to learn how to see. At least the market in Mehanna was a colorful one. Every Thursday, people from a variety of ethnic groups converged on Mehanna to buy and sell. Tall, angular Fulani women sold butter and curdled milk. Bearing salt tablets from deep in the Sahara, nomadic Tuaregs, wrapped in blue and black turbans that veiled their mouths, arrived atop their camels. Hausa men from the eastern region of Niger butchered meat and sold leather goods. Songhay people from islands in the Niger River brought vegetables, tobacco, and fish.

As it turned out, my trip to Mehanna enabled me to learn more about divination than I had anticipated. At the market I saw a friend, Fatouma Seyni, who asked me to visit her house late one afternoon. After we drank tea and chatted, Fatouma told me that she was a diviner.

"The shells say that I should teach you about divination," she informed me.

The path of divination had opened for me—at least partially. I took lessons from her. She taught me configurations that indicated sickness, death. She showed me how to detect the presence of a witch, the loss of money, and the arrival of good fortune—either riches, or good health after a bout of sickness. She taught me how to see a "path that was blocked" and to divine what might be blocking the path. She pointed out how to see trouble on a person's path. After helping me to learn a little bit about reading shells, she abruptly dismissed me. "You've learned enough for now. You'll be back. I've seen it in the shells. When you return, we'll continue."

"Is that the wish of the King of the Sky?" I asked.

"Of course," she said enthusiastically. "The shells are power. If you move forward too fast or read them too often, they will make you sick. When I read them too much I get headaches."

Reluctantly, I did as she asked and returned to Tillaberi to say my farewells to Adamu Jenitongo. Before leaving Niger that year, I threw shells for several associates in Niamey, Niger's capital city. I saw configurations, but couldn't figure out a point of reference. I could see sickness and good fortune but didn't know how to attribute them to a particular person. I had not yet heard Wambata's voice.

❀ ❀ ❀

The development of my vision has been a slow process. As the years have progressed I have learned more about a seemingly infinite array of shell configurations. Ten years after first studying with Adamu Jenitongo, I began to sense Wambata's voice during divination sessions for friends and family. That gentle breeze of a voice would give me a point of reference in shell configurations, which enabled me to make better sense of the patterns. I gained some ability to see and hear the past, present, and future. My path, as Adamu Jenitongo would have said, had opened. This development encouraged me to throw shells more regularly. My enthusiasm, though, exacted a price, for like my teacher Fatouma Seyni, this turn of events also gave me severe headaches. When I became more circumspect about throwing shells, the headaches disappeared. The experience reminded me once again that one should learn about sorcery in a deliberate and respectful way. The shells have taught me a number of important lessons about living life in the contemporary world. Sorcerers cannot master shells, as the Songhay would phrase it, unless they have mastered themselves. Such mastery means that sorcerers need to know themselves, to again evoke the ideas of Antonin Artaud, with a cruel honestly. As this emotionally painful self-vision ripens with age, so does the capacity to read the past, present, and future. Following this path, the sorcerer learns to see as well as look, to hear as well as listen.

Twenty-five years ago, Djibo Mounmouni said to me: "You look but you don't see. You listen but you don't hear. You touch but you don't feel." Although my abilities cannot be compared with those of Adamu Jenitongo or Fatouma Seyni, I have slowly and deliberately tried to develop my capacity to see and hear. When my path unexpectedly led me into the village of the sick, these sensibilities deepened. When I stepped into the world of cancer and experienced blood tests, CAT scans, bone-marrow biopsies, and the cool surge of chemotherapy drugs in my blood, I understood more fully what it meant to feel.

The sorcerous notion of vision may seem to have little connection to the world of cancer. Before becoming a cancer patient, I considered divination a powerful tool that sorcerers use to diagnose illnesses and to anticipate trouble along the life path. Divination now seems similar to screening tests that physicians employ to detect lung, breast, or colon cancer or to compute the probability of developing prostate or cervical cancer. The issue with these screening tests—and divination—is whether you need or want to know what the future holds. There has been a great deal of debate about medical screening. Many physicians advocate regular procedures (mammograms, Pap smears, and colonoscopies) and various blood tests, like the prostate-specific antigen (PSA), to screen for cancers. Other physicians question the usefulness of many of these procedures and tests.[6]

American culture is an exceedingly optimistic one.[7] We expect good news. We prize people with sunny dispositions. We accentuate the positive. We avoid discussion or acknowledgment of serious illness. If you are ignorant of trouble, we reason, you are freed from its burdens. The prospect of death is frightening. In mainstream American culture, as sociologist Arthur Frank argues in his noteworthy book *The Wounded Storyteller,* a lack of optimism leads to pessimism. Pessimism then leads to alienation, which in turn leads to a lack of well-being, which in the end makes us sick. If you get something as insidious as cancer, it must be your fault: you smoked too much, you exposed yourself to too much sunlight, or you repressed your emotions, which weakened your immune system.

Cancer presents a profound cultural challenge. Because cancer is a set of disintegrative diseases that implicate blood, bowels, bone, and organs, elements we also avoid discussing in polite society, some of us whisper or avoid saying the word *cancer*—especially if its long arm has touched us directly or indirectly. As Susan Sontag brilliantly portrayed in her book *Illness as Metaphor,* cancer is perceived as an evil. As such it shares many similarities with African conceptions of witchcraft. In West African societies, you avoid discussion of witches. When you talk about a witch, it is usually in a whisper or in a foreign language. Human beings walk in the daylight; witches dwell in the night. A person's identity and wealth are usually acquired through the father's blood. Witches usually receive their nefarious power through mother's milk. Like African witchcraft, cancer is the underside of our culture, the antithesis of what we want to exist. Even so, every person has the potential to develop cancer. Our bodies routinely produce cancerous cells that our immune systems routinely destroy.[8] Cancer is not only the underside of our culture but also the hidden dimension of our bodies.

When lymphoma cells produced a bulky tumor in my abdomen, I realized that we all live with cancer. It implicates everyone in one way or another. Before my diagnosis, my experience as a student of sorcery, which was admittedly limited, convinced me that my body was a fortress. Because the men in my family had led healthy lives well into old age, I thought that I would also enjoy good health as I aged. On rare occasions when I reflected about cancer, my thinking conformed to the poorly informed notion of many other people in the village of the healthy in which good health is taken for granted: namely, that cancer developed in other people, especially those with self-destructive habits. How could cancer affect me?

The thought of cancer never really entered my consciousness until Brian Markson, during a routine physical, felt an "un-

defined mass" in my abdomen. That event changed my life forever and focused my vision. Cancer compelled me to see myself—my being—more clearly. The central component of the
vision of Songhay sorcerers, I now understood, concentrated not
so much on past, present, and future, but on seeing things clearly.
This revelation reduced my physical and emotional isolation in
the world of cancer. It provided me comfort in uncomfortable
circumstances.

❊   ❊   ❊

Developing the capacity to see things clearly raises the issue of
how realistic we should be. Should you be optimistic or pessimistic about the future? Americans tend to be optimists. Even
after the shock and horror of the September 11 terrorist attacks,
an ABC–*Washington Post* poll about the aftermath of the attacks
indicated that the majority of Americans remained optimistic
about the future. Eight of every ten respondents reported a
hopeful outlook for the future.[9] As embodied in the sunny dis-
position of President Ronald Reagan, optimism is an essential
aspect of mainstream American culture. Millions of Americans
it seems to me share this optimism; they feel—or have felt—that
nothing can do them real harm. By the same token, millions of
Americans are pessimistic about the future. Suspicious of trouble lurking in every square inch of her world, my grandmother
took extraordinary measures to protect herself from the world's
evils.

Social psychologists like Martin Seligman, author of the
1991 book *Learned Optimism,* have conducted extensive research
on the benefits of an optimistic view of the world. In the past
many psychologists argued that an optimistic worldview provided greater emotional and physical well-being than one riven
with pessimism. According to Seligman and others, optimism,
which can be learned, enables people to live longer, healthier,

and happier lives, as compared with the experience of pessimistic people. Pessimism can lead to a sense of helplessness and trigger depression. Helplessness and depression, in turn, weaken the immune system, priming the body for serious illnesses and even premature death. In studies of cancer patients, for example, researchers have found that pessimism is an important risk factor in cancer mortality in people under the age of sixty.[10] This set of assumptions seems to have diffused into widespread folk wisdom about how pessimism, repressed desire, and depressive tendencies enable cancer to invade weakened body defenses.

More recently a few psychologists have argued that a degree of pessimism is a good thing. They suggest that overly optimistic people are ill prepared for misfortune or serious illness. When a serious illness like cancer strikes, the worlds of overly optimistic people are completely overturned. To adapt to this unexpected turn of events, they may deny the seriousness of their illness or become embittered. In Arthur Frank's 1991 book, *At the Will of the Body*, in which the author describes his own struggles with cancer and heart disease, Frank recounts the story of another cancer patient who, before being diagnosed, was an optimist. Before he had developed leukemia in his early fifties, this person enjoyed sports, dining, and traveling. He couldn't believe that someone in such excellent physical condition could develop cancer. Following a course of chemotherapy, the man went into remission, but could not help feeling bitter about his fate. He became reclusive and resentful. Despite the absence of symptoms, he refused to enjoy his life. His remission lasted three years. As he lay dying, he finally realized that he had wasted the last good years of his life. He died with regret.[11] Had his early optimism ultimately undermined his will to live?

This thinking on the repercussions of a person's view of the world does not suggest that a person should either dispense with optimism or embrace pessimism. Rather, it suggests that we should attempt, like the Songhay sorcerer, to see things clearly. Being optimistic should not blind us from reality. It suggests that you can be pessimistic, but not in a way that clouds your vision completely. Above all, you should attempt to be prepared to confront whatever life presents—pragmatic optimism laced with a practical pessimism.

When Joel Rubin announced that I had lymphoma, the news shattered my optimistic, relatively trouble-free life. How could I, of all people, have lymphoma?

"We don't know the cause," he stated in one of his conversations with me. "Maybe it's environmental. It might be genetic. We really don't know." There was evidently no explanation of how I had developed lymphoma. In these circumstances, it is impossible to avoid the question "Why me?"

When I got the bad news, I tried not to dwell on these imponderables. I did not return home, take out my cowry shells, and attempt to "see" who or what had caused my illness. I did not try to see the date of my death. Like Songhay sorcerers, I attempted to see things—including myself—more clearly. I attempted to prepare myself for what had appeared on my path. I read widely about my illness and possible treatments for it. To keep myself going, I tried to eat well and get plenty of sleep. I continued to write and do my work. I tried to enjoy my life. Although these measures did not wash away my worries about pain and death, they did sustain me through eight months of chemotherapy. They sustain me now that I'm in remission. And yet, like Songhay sorcerers, I realize that in the future I will face trouble for which I must be prepared. If the medical literature is accurate, it is only a matter of time until lymphoma cells reappear in my body. When that happens I will have to undergo more diagnostic tests and more treatments.[12] Despite the "darkness" of my future, I hope that my tempered optimism will enable me to enjoy the pleasures of good health for as long as I can.

❀ ❀ ❀

Among the Songhay, clear vision also embodies a sense of humility, which is yet another important component of Songhay sorcery that can be useful to cancer patients. Arrogance, I have learned, can do a person great harm. This notion is especially relevant to people confronting serious illness. As David Napier describes in his book *The Age of Immunology* (2003), the medical stance toward illness is militaristic. Illness is an invading force, a foreigner attempting to colonize the body. That alien force must first be subdued and then eliminated. Medical science has developed an impressive array of technological weapons to kill invading cells, bacteria and viruses, which leads to the belief that we have the capacity to eradicate illnesses like cancer. This notion solidifies the ideology in the village of the healthy: namely, that illness is a temporary nuisance that can be quickly and totally cured. In Balinese and Songhay society, by contrast, people have a more humble take on illness. Having to live with inadequate medical care, they are compelled to respect the power of illness, which means that they attempt to incorporate it into their lives. If illness is incorporated into one's life, people can use it to become stronger in body and wiser in spirit.

In Songhay and Balinese society, then, the specter of disease prompts most people to take a humble approach to illness. If my case is at all typical, the pill of humility is a difficult one for many Americans to swallow. In 1984, after having fled Wanzerbé in fear for my life, I decided to learn from several herbalists I had met in Niger's capital city, Niamey. Trying to put Wanzerbé behind me, I now divided time between the Niamey herbalists and Adamu Jenitongo, from whom I hoped to learn more about sorcerous plants.

In Niamey, I passed the days with herbalist friends in a space shaded by acacias and eucalyptus tress. This spot was adjacent to a paved road that separated Niamey's frenetic fish and vegetable market from a line of shops housed in cement buildings. Across the street the din of shoppers buying and selling dried tomatoes, bananas, oranges, whole and powdered hot peppers, peanut cakes, and fresh, fly-covered meat echoed in the dry air. Breezes carried the pungent odor of fresh and dried Niger River fish. Behind us, people wandered in and out of the shops. Exposure to sun, dust, and sand gave the whitewashed building facades a dull brown hue.

Herbalists had long been setting up shop at this interstice of traditional and modern economic life. This was the place where they had unrolled their mats to display their products— assortments of resins, roots, stems, barks, and leaves either tied in small bundles or molded into small mounds. Some of the herbalists put out dried snakeskin, dried bird carcasses, and lizard skulls. Sorcerers use these animal elements to make amulets or to concoct *kusu,* the food of power.

The most senior herbalist, Soumana Yacouba, insisted that I spend my days seated next to him. He was a short, muscular man, perhaps fifty years old, who had been gathering and selling herbs for more than thirty years. He loved to tell stories. Continuous contact with dust had clouded his deep-set brown eyes. A tribal scar cut across his left cheek. A short, neatly trimmed beard framed his square face. Unlike Adamu Jenitongo, whose people were Songhay from Wanzerbé, Soumana Yacouba's folk lived in a small village that bordered the Niger River. Whereas Adamu Jenitongo's magic and healing capacities had been passed down from the great Songhay king, Sonni Ali Ber (1463–1491), Soumana Yacouba's knowledge originated from a long line of river sorcerers. Masters of the river, called *Do* in Songhay, had the ability to spend long periods of time under water. They were said to be "of the water," and many of their most potent medicines came from the depths of the Niger River.

Every morning I would bring Soumana Yacouba breakfast

and sit down next to him. We would spend much of the day comparing the efficacy of plants and manufactured medicines. He found "French" medicines too expensive and of limited value in the treatment of many African conditions. He claimed to have effective medicines for dysentery, both amoebic and bacterial, asthma, syphilis, gonorrhea, malaria, tropical ulcers, and hepatitis. He taught me how to recognize specific African conditions and how to mix herbal cocktails to treat them. We talked at length about life in America and life along the Niger River. I told Soumana about how my ancestors had come from eastern Europe just before World War I. He recounted the story of his family, which had lived along the same bend in the Niger River for more than eight hundred years. He couldn't understand how people in America—or anywhere else—could live alone. I had difficulty accepting his belief that his people had evolved from a large round-headed Niger River fish, called *desi*. These fish have red flesh, whiskers, and long tentacles that emerge from their heads. They can submerge into the mud of a drying water hole and survive for months.

One bright and clear December morning I brought Soumana Yacouba a bowl of warm milk and several baguettes. We dipped pieces of bread into the milk and savored the rich flavor. Although vendors had begun to fill up the spaces in the vegetable market, no one had stopped by to buy medicinal plants. Shoppers hadn't yet arrived at the shops.

"I love cool, crisp days in the cold season," Soumana stated. "It's a good time to harvest plants. In a few days, I will go off to the countryside to find plants. My younger brother will come here." He took kola nuts from the pocket of his black drawstring trousers. "It is a good time," he reiterated.

A tall, thickly built woman walked up to our spot. She wore an indigo homespun wraparound skirt with a matching top and headscarf. "My greetings to you both," she said. Her smile revealed many missing teeth.

We returned her greetings.

"The cold has given me rheumatism," she complained. "My legs are stiff. So is my back."

Soumana turned to me. "What is the problem?" he asked, always the teacher.

"She has a cool illness," I said.

"And how can we help her?" he asked.

I picked up a bundle of *zam turi* barks, which had the hue of red clay. "Will these work?"

Soumana nodded. "Tell the woman what to do," he said.

"Madam," I said, excited to be of help to someone "You first must pulverize the bark. Then add three pinches of it to coffee, hot milk, or hot water. Let the mixture cool a bit and then drink it. Do this each morning until the cool illness goes away."

Soumana said nothing. The woman nodded. I handed her the bundle of bark. She pulled out a small satchel from under her skirt and took out fifty francs (twenty cents). "Is that enough, sir?" she asked Soumana.

Soumana took the money and said nothing. As the woman walked away, he turned toward me. "You did well." He produced more kola and put it into his mouth.

I felt a sense of pride.

"Even though I'm getting older and know the plants of the bush and the river, my time has not yet come," Soumana said unexpectedly.

"What do you mean?" I asked.

"The great secrets of our folk have not been revealed to me. I'm not ready." He took a deep breath. "Before my mother dies, she will tell me the important things. Only then."

"That's difficult," I observed with my Western impatience.

"No," he retorted. "My time will come."

Just then a young man appeared in front of us. He was dressed in a nicely tailored brown Sahelian suit, a pair of trousers matched with an overhanging shirt with two flap pockets over the chest. He carried a clipboard and pen.

"I'm a medical student," he announced, "I've been doing research on herbal medicine and I—"

"Do you not greet people when you first see them?" Soumana interrupted.

The young man took a step back and hugged his clipboard. "How goes the morning?" he asked. Confident that he had given a proper greeting, he continued. "I am a medical student, studying the plants that herbalists prescribe. I want to collect plants that are used to treat disease."

Soumana offered him a kola nut

"Thank you, I don't chew." He looked closely at his clipboard. "I've already collected about ten plants. Do you have *sabaara*?"

"You mean the plant that has ninety-nine different uses?" Soumana turned to me. "Paul, have you seen any *sabaara*?" he asked, giving me a conspiratorial wink.

I looked at Soumana's display. "No."

Soumana looked at the medical student. "I'm sorry. We don't have any. If you go to the Bukoki market, you might find it." He turned toward me. "What do you think?"

"The Hausa herbalists there might have some," I stated.

Without saying farewell, the medical student left.

I picked up a bundle of *sabaara*. "Why didn't you give him what he was looking for?"

Soumana frowned. "I didn't like him. You come here every day. You understand what respect is. He comes here for the first time, does not even greet us, and wants to know the secrets of my heritage. You must earn knowledge. To earn it, misfortune must test your courage. Knowledge is greater than we are. You have to learn it slowly. You have to respect its power."

※ ※ ※

Rather than learning from Soumana's admonitions about impatience and respect, I developed over the course of our sessions a potentially dangerous hubris. Memories of paralysis and death in Wanzerbé receded to the background of my consciousness. I was no longer on "the path of power," I reasoned, and had little to fear from the spite of other sorcerers. On the "path of plants," knowledge and practice seemed more concrete—better suited to my view of the world. I began to collect medicinal herbs. I used them to treat my own minor medical problems, and I gave them to friends and told them how to prepare tonics or salves. I also prepared herbal mixtures that enabled people to face their foes with grit and determination. Having learned from people like Adamu Jenitongo and Soumana Yacouba, I felt that my skills in plant sorcery had increased exponentially.

In retrospect, I continue to be surprised about how selective a person's perception can be. When I began my studies with Soumana Yacouba, I had been an apprentice sorcerer for more than eight years. I had committed to memory scores of sorcerous incantations. I had identified hundreds of medicinal and sorcerous plants. I had mixed medicinal tonics and sorcerous potions for dozens of people. In the configurations of cowry shells, I had seen bits of the past, present, and future. Despite this record of accomplishment, I had been quite blind to the central principles of Songhay sorcery—principles that my teachers articulated regularly through words and practice.

Consider the *genji how.* I had recited the first few lines of it hundreds of times, but had not fully understood their meaning. Those lines trace the genealogy of power. Power, according to Songhay beliefs, comes from N'debbi, the intermediary between the High God and human beings. N'debbi gave power to the people of the past, who passed it down from generation to generation until it reached contemporary practitioners. "What was in their minds," according to the text, "is in my mind. "What was in their lips is in my lips. What was in their hearts is in my heart." The genealogical significance of the passage was immediately apparent. What I didn't realize until I confronted cancer was that I, like all people who tried to practice healing, was but a trickle in the stream of sorcery.

Among the Songhay people, sorcery had existed thousands of years before my birth and will continue to be practiced long after my death. A Songhay sorcerer's contribution to society is but a small moment in the flow of history. The struggle of sorcerers, I have slowly come to realize, is to situate themselves in the sweep of history, adjust to it, practice what they have learned, refine their knowledge, and then pass it on to the next generation.

This orientation, like that of sorcerous vision, presents a cultural challenge to many Americans. I suggested earlier that while our characteristic sense of unbridled optimism is usually a very positive personal quality, it could be harmful when we face a serious illness like cancer. In the same vein, the sorcerous conception that you are a very small element in the broad flow of history runs counter to our sense of individualism, which can also be harmful when a person confronts serious illness.

There are many examples of how individualism influences our everyday life. When we get into a buffet line we usually take food for our individual consumption. Our focus is usually a personal one. In similar circumstances, many Songhay would limit their food selection to copious amounts of one food, bread, corn, or chicken, which they would place in the middle of a table for group consumption. In Songhay villages, as in many towns throughout the world, food is prepared for and consumed by a group, which is one example of how Songhay orient themselves toward the group.

Consider just how "personal" we tend to be. We have personal income and personal trainers. We attempt to "personalize" our lives. We have personal computers with individual passwords. We can even customize our computers to make them even more personalized. When talk gets serious, we get "personal," because we are talking about matters that really matter—to us as individuals. We amass personal possessions that, upon death, we bequeath to family and friends, following the dictates of our individual desires as stated in a last will and testament.

We are taught that hard work brings success—financial reward, personal possessions, and personal recognition. This cultural orientation often compels us to think that we are in control of our lives. We fill in personal planners. We set personal objectives. The professionals who hire us, who are sometimes called "human resources specialists," work in personnel. Whatever we call them, these specialists deal with "personal relations." Important interview questions usually include: "What are your objectives for the next five years? What goals will you have met in ten years?" These questions imply that if you are strong and self-reliant, you can shape your life and control your destiny. People who fit these "strong" parameters, which are shaped by optimism, get hired and quickly move up the ladder of success in mainstream American institutions: government, corporations, and universities. These cultural themes tend to reinforce notions of individualism and reduce our willingness to respect that which is different, including, of course, a (different) set of malignant cells growing in your body. In the end, our more individualistic orientation toward social life also contributes to the idea that through personal action we can conquer nature, including, of course, illnesses like cancer.

I don't mean to imply that mainstream Americans have no sense of the group. We do. Families are a primary resource of social support in America. In tough times many people turn to their families for financial assistance and emotional reinforcement. Even though our families provide us with much-needed reinforcement, that support, in contrast to social support in more collectivist societies, is usually directed toward the pursuit of individual interests and the achievement of personal goals. Team sports are another case in point of how groups tend to reinforce individual pursuits in America. In contemporary American culture, we value the team player. No matter the degree of individual achievement, team players play for the good of the team; they may even sacrifice the spotlight of individual attention to maintain team harmony. In corporate culture, which is often closely allied to that of team sports, employees are also urged to be "team players." Good team playing, it is argued, helps to control corporate destiny, which, in turn, enhances corporate profitably. Given the philosophy of trickle-down economics, corporate profitably benefits everybody. The underside of trickle-down profitability in corporations, of course, is that it benefits some people more than it does others. By the same token, in professional sports some team players are given higher salaries than others are. In other words, the ultimate goal of team playing in sports or in corporations is individual advancement based upon "personal" performance. Despite these collective tendencies in team sports and corporate culture, the individual remains central to mainstream American social relations, which has a profound impact on how patients, caregivers, physicians, nurses, and medical institutions conceive of and respond to serious illnesses like cancer. It is not easy to chart a course toward humility in contemporary mainstream American culture.

Many peoples of the world, including, of course, the Songhay, construct social relations very differently. As already mentioned, they focus more on the group than on the individual. This tendency has an impact on most aspects of their lives, including how they respond to serious illnesses. In most Songhay villages, for example, families rather than individuals possess property. Families "own" land and livestock, which is passed down "in the family" from generation to generation. Individual accomplishment in business or government brings with it not only money and possessions, but the obligation to share resources with less accomplished family members. On payday the relatives of Nigerien civil servants invariably descend upon them, often from great distances, to demand their share of the family member's salary. By the end of the payday blood kin have often consumed much of the civil servants' money.[13]

In Mehanna, the village where I conducted my early fieldwork, a civil servant complained continuously about his family. As the only salaried member of his kindred, he sent much of his monthly stipend to his parents and siblings. Due to his relative isolation in Mehanna, he had managed to keep a bit of money for himself. He had even managed to buy a powerful shortwave radio, which we would listen to in the evening. One evening I paid him a visit, but did not hear the radio—a customary evening sound in his compound.

"Where's the radio, Moussa?" I asked.

"My older brother came for a visit," he said with resignation. "He wanted the radio." Moussa shrugged his shoulders. "I had to give it to him."

For many Songhay, as for many peoples in the world, success is not only measured in how much wealth you can acquire, but also in how much of it you are able to give away. The ideal image of an accomplished person among the Songhay would be a businessman or civil servant who, despite impressive wealth, lives modestly because he or she shares his income with family members.

I had been taught that generosity is admirable. Indeed, the wealthiest Americans often become philanthropists who give away much of their money. Even so, American philanthropists rarely deny themselves a possession in the name of self-denying philanthropy. Bill Gates has given away millions of dollars, but does not live modestly. Generosity is admirable, but it has limits.

What, then, is the payoff for a Songhay whose generosity results in self-denial? It may come from an increased measure of respect. We usually accord a healthy respect to people who have amassed fortunes. This wealth is usually measured in dollars. Although peoples like the Songhay certainly don't ignore a person's worth in dollars, they also measure "wealth in people." For them the question is not only "how much am I worth?" but also "how many people are in my network?" We respect individuals who have acquired great wealth, who have obtained some kind of celebrity, or who, like physicians, occupy prestigious social positions. In Songhay culture, great respect is accorded to people who, through acts of self-denial, are able to maintain good relations in a variety of personal networks. A man who has wealth in people will never be abandoned socially or emotionally, for the individuals in his network will provide him continuous comfort and support.

This more collective view of the world also implicates the possession of knowledge. Among many African peoples, knowledge, like wealth in people, is a precious commodity. It is not something that an individual owns; rather, it is something that one masters, refines, and passes along. West African griots fit into this category. As bards, they commit to memory long epic poems that chronicle the past. Griots are the embodiment of West African history. They are masters of old words. And yet, griots do not "own" the old words they have mastered; the old words own them. Humbled by the forces of history, they become intermediaries between past and present. Griots might refine the telling of an epic, but would never change its narrative structure or manipulate its meaning. By consuming history, griots are consumed by it. Extending this formula to contemporary North American social life, what can we say about how medical professionals approach knowledge? Do they master it, creating a state of certitude that leads to arrogance, or does medical knowledge master them, creating a state of incertitude that leads to humility?

Like physicians, sorcerers heal the sick, but their approach to knowledge reflects a more collectivist orientation that usually leads to a humble and respectful approach to illness and healing. Sorcerers are the embodiment of power. They are the masters of incantations, plants, and magic. And yet, sorcerers, do not own this power; the power owns them. It is said that in the process of eating power, in the form of the aforementioned *kusu*, sorcerers are consumed by power. Particular sorcerers may become accomplished practitioners who attract clients from far and wide, but no matter their renown, the collective power of "those who came before" restrains their sense of self. In this way the sorcerer is part of a larger tradition of sorcery. Traditions of the past constrain an individual's will in the present. The precedents of the past set the parameters within which sorcerers learn, practice, and refine power. By the same token, these precedents underscore the limits of the individual sorcerer's power as well as his obligation to pass power on to the next generation. Sorcery, then, is far more powerful than any sorcerer is. This set of time-honored principles leads one on a path from youthful arrogance to seasoned humility.

❅   ❅   ❅

Like sorcery, cancer charts a course toward humility. Cancer propels you down a difficult path on which it is important to be humble. If you are arrogant about life and believe that you can master illness, a disease, like cancer, can force you into a needlessly desperate corner. The onset of many cancers is sometimes sudden and often without symptoms. Take the case of a sixty-five-year-old man who was recently diagnosed with terminal colorectal cancer. Until just before his diagnosis, he led an active life. He exercised regularly, played golf, looked after his semi-ambulatory wife, and participated often in family outings. From a mainstream American perspective, he led an exemplary life, a life of which he could be proud. At a routine physical his doctor pronounced him "fit." This pronouncement gave him—and his family—a sense of assurance about the future. Toward the end of the year, however, he experienced fatigue and flu-like symptoms. He went to see his physician, who scheduled him for diagnostic tests. The results of these tests showed a baseball-size tumor in his colon that had metastasized. Malignant tumors had colonized his liver and had appeared in swollen lymph nodes throughout his body. One tumor, which had attached itself to the artery leading to the brain, had restricted blood flow to that part of his body. The man's oncologist estimated that the colorectal tumor had been silently developing for ten years. He gave the man a dim prognosis: two weeks to six months to live.

This story is an all too common one in contemporary life. A healthy, active person who exhibits few, if any, symptoms, is told that she or he has cancer, a pronouncement that in the minds of many people is usually the equivalent of a death sentence. Optimism fades and feelings of control over one's life dissipate. Fear appears and helplessness fills the void created by a confrontation with death. Fear and helplessness can trigger depression, which often develops after a cancer diagnosis.[14] Life spins even more out of control as we worry about a painful and premature death.

No formula can wash away the pain and suffering that comes with the diagnosis and treatment of cancer. For many people, denial can have short-term effectiveness. For others, faith, spirituality, and ritual can provide a degree of solace. Support groups can decrease the cancer patient's isolation. In a support group you are more likely to say what you feel and take comfort through commiseration with others who more or less share your fate. Even so, can participation in support groups deflect powerful themes that culturally disadvantage cancer patients? Perhaps they can to some extent. But can they alter the general perception that cancer is evil, that cancer changes social relationships, that cancer makes life spin out of control? As I indicated earlier, no matter the degree of support that they have, cancer patients, like the African sorcerer, must confront their illness alone.

Such a lonely assessment is by no means a prescription for hopeless pain and suffering. On the contrary, a sense of humility can put pain and suffering into a context larger than the personal. This view is the one that most Songhay people hold. Illness is always lurking. Like the High God and the spirits, the force of illness is greater than any individual is. Illness is part of life; it lies within us and waits for the right moment to appear. The ideal for Songhay, especially Songhay sorcerers, is to learn to respect the unalterable presence of illness and live with it. Songhay sorcerers believe that if you learn to live with illness, your being becomes stronger and stronger.

Like the notions of pragmatic pessimism, the idea of living with an illness runs counter to major themes in American culture. No one wants to live with an illness. If we contract an illness, we want to conquer it. Illnesses are metaphorically framed, as is medical discourse, in terms of war. We are at war with disease. We fight infection. Bacteria invade our bodies and colonize our cells. Our immune systems produce natural killer cells that ambush the invaders so that we can win our battle with illness.

The world of cancer is particularly fraught with war metaphors. We are fighting the war on cancer. Cancer cells attack and overwhelm healthy cells. They slowly and inexorably grow and overwhelm the opposition—our body's natural defenses. When cancer first appears technicians run reconnaissance tests that pinpoint the enemy's position and describe the enemy's internal arsenal of defenses. Oncologists then send a sortie of chemotherapy agents on search-and-destroy missions. These agents destroy the enemy, but also kill healthy bystanders—collateral damage. These missions often result in heavy casualties. If you live through this campaign, though, you become known as a veteran, a survivor. Survivors then tell "war" stories to help other foot soldiers in the war effort.

In military culture, one is taught to follow orders. Lack of obedience and a state of disorder create inefficiency and weakness. Illness also creates "disorders." There are neurological disorders, gastrointestinal disorders, and, of course, psychological disorders. As in military culture, disorders are culturally unacceptable in mainstream American culture. We therefore engage in monumental efforts to order our disorders through frontal attack. We are encouraged to change our diets and moderate our drinking. We pay billions of dollars annually to ingest millions of over-the-counter and prescription drugs. We sometimes agree to cosmetic, minor, or major surgery. But can we bring order to the chaos of life? I once thought so, but living in the village of the sick has made me more respectful of the disorder of social life. It has also shown me that if you respect illness, you can use it to develop your being.

※ ※ ※

Adamu Jenitongo once asked to look at the medical supplies I brought with me to Niger. I had a plastic container filled with bandages, topical creams, antimalarial tablets, and antacids. A stool-sample kit could confirm a case of amoebic dysentery. A small vial of iodine tablets could secure water from any source.

"Why did you bring so many pills?" he asked. "What if you got something that is stronger than the pills?"

"Then I'd go to the hospital or leave and go back to America for treatment."

"And what if you got something that they couldn't cure at hospital or in America?"

"Then I'd die," I said, feeling that such an event would be unlikely.

"Exactly so," he proclaimed without further elaboration.

For many years I paid little attention to this exchange. Having experienced a life-threatening disease like cancer, I finally understood what Adamu Jenitongo wanted to teach me so many years ago. Although the technological marvels of modern medicine may make you the survivor of many battles, can you ever win the war?

Adamu Jenitongo told me that one needs to respect illness as a part of life. Individuals should treat their illnesses and seek health and vitality. By the same token, the restoration of health does not make you a conqueror. For someone like Adamu Jenitongo, an individual is but a trickle in life's stream. We all live on borrowed time. We should, following the wisdom of Adamu Jenitongo, make the most of our borrowed time. To accomplish this feat, he would say, we need to pick our battles very carefully and exert our force when it is important to do so. This strategy defines the Songhay sorcerer's notion of courage.

❀ ❀ ❀

In Songhay philosophy, internal and external harmony enables a person to see life more clearly. During one of my research trips to Niger to study Songhay religion, I headed for the small town of Tillaberi and Adamu Jenitongo's dune-top compound. My trip to Tillaberi went smoothly. Thankfully, we didn't run out of gas or hear the pop and thump of a flat tire. The regular driver had given up drinking, which meant that his speed wasn't too excessive. Given his sobriety, he negotiated the fearsomely narrow "bridge of death" with great finesse. That day the police seemed uninterested in inspections. To add to this good fortune, three young boys happened to be at the Tillaberi bus depot to help me carry my gear across the dunes to Adamu Jenitongo's. I had come bearing gifts for Adamu Jenitongo, his two wives, and his two sons. Moru, the younger son, put my gear in the spirit hut and I prepared for what I thought would be an important stint of field research.

Adamu Jenitongo gave me "vision" that year. He also taught me about farming magic and talked extensively about the spirits in the Songhay pantheon. At night we slept peacefully in the spirit hut amid ritual objects, some new, some old. In the mornings, I would build a small fire to warm our aching bones and boil water for coffee—freeze-dried Nescafé mixed with sweetened evaporated milk.

One night I learned another lesson that I would remember

years later, when I was forced to deal with cancer. Just before dawn Adamu Jenitongo shook me gently. In the fuzzy world between sleep and consciousness, I saw him put his finger to his lips. Was I dreaming? He tugged at my arm and motioned for me to get up slowly. He came close to me. "Snake," he whispered.

My eyes widened. He put his hand over my mouth. "Be quiet," he whispered. "I know what to do." He found a hard wood baton and slowly lifted the corner of his straw sleeping mat. A viper had slipped under Adamu Jenitongo's mat. It had coiled itself and appeared to be asleep. In a lightning-quick move, he bashed in the snake's head. He then picked it up and brought it outside. Holding it up, he shook his head. "The world is spoiled. The world is spoiled."

"What do you mean, *Baba*?" I asked, puzzled.

"Someone sent this snake to bite me," he answered calmly. "They are jealous of me. They wish to harm me. They'd like to see me die."

"How could someone send a snake to bite only you?"

He laughed. "You still have much to learn, my son," he said. "There are many people who can control the movement of snakes." He paused and smiled, revealing several incisors that tooth decay had reduced to little more than blackened stumps. "There is medicine that calms snakes." He paused once again for effect. "A snake has never bitten me."

"Do you know who sent the viper?" I asked.

"Of course," he said, chuckling. "I know who sent it."

"What will you do?"

"He's sent many snakes, my son. He'll send others."

"But aren't you concerned that a snake might bite one of your wives or children?"

"They're protected."

I couldn't comprehend his nonchalance. "But shouldn't this person be punished?"

"A younger sorcerer might try to make him sick, or even kill him, but I have chosen to ignore his efforts." He paused a moment. "A true sorcerer must not waste energy on needless battles. You must avoid conflict as often as possible. When you do fight a battle, make sure it is an important one. Knowing when not to fight is the mark of courage; it prepares you for battles worthy of your power."

These words remained lodged in the recesses of my mind until I confronted cancer, which changed many things in my life, including my grasp of the sorcerer's conception of courage. Here was an entity, as Adamu Jenitongo might say, worthy of my respectful attention. In some ways, cancer has guided me back to sorcery's path, and focused my energies on a relationship with a powerful force. I began to see how sorcery could help Songhay people to struggle with the powerful forces of their world. In due course, I finally began to understand what courage entailed.

❀ ❀ ❀

In the waiting and infusion rooms of The Cancer Center, memories of Adamu Jenitongo served as my guide and his wisdom once again gave me the courage and strength to confront difficult circumstances. The courage of several fellow cancer patients also inspired me. At The Cancer Center I met people who, despite their emotional and physical pain, carried themselves with quiet dignity. Rarely did I hear them complain to others about their fate. Rarely did I hear them raise their voices in anger. Instead I saw people trying to enjoy music, absorb themselves in a book, or make plans with a family member or friend.

I remember one woman in the infusion room who, judging from the thickness of her file, had long been a cancer patient. She was tall, overweight, and dressed in loose-fitting khaki slacks and a short-sleeve plaid blouse that revealed a grotesquely swollen left arm. Her treatment had resulted in lymphedema, a retention of lymph fluids that produces localized swelling—not an uncommon condition for some cancer patients. She wore a scarf to cover her baldness.

One of the oncology nurses carried tubes and medicine over to her recliner, which was next to mine. "How are you doing today?" the nurse asked warmly.

"Not too bad," the woman replied.

She touched the swollen arm. "Is it causing you pain?" the nurse asked.

"It's really not too bad," the woman answered, composed.

"That's good," the nurse replied. "Can we take a look at your catheter?" she asked. "I have to make sure it's clean." The nurse examined a catheter that had been surgically inserted into the woman's chest. When cancer patients receive frequent and massive doses of chemotherapy drugs, surgeons insert catheters. "Clean" catheters protect the integrity of the patient's veins and enable efficient flow of chemotherapy drugs into the body. "It looks good."

"I try to keep it clean," the woman said.

The nurse attached the line and administered the drug. "Are you going to be okay?" she asked the woman.

"I'll be fine," the woman said. Moments later she had fallen asleep.

This woman's calm and strong manner impressed me immensely. If I faced similar circumstances, I wondered, could I confront them with such courage? She must have been in great emotional and physical pain. She seemed to have accepted her state with dignity and wanted, or so it seemed to me, to get on with her life. From the perspective of Songhay sorcery, this woman had perhaps learned how to see clearly and walk on her path with pragmatic confidence.

From the vantage of the Songhay, this woman could be seen as someone who had stood up to her illness and engaged it with quiet strength and determination. Winning, I have come to realize, is not the goal of everyday confrontations. Cancer patients, old and young, male and female, have often learned to live with their illness and accept the difficult fact that death is part of life. Those lessons have enabled them to maintain their dignity and improve the quality of their lives. For me, that is the mark of courage, the courage of the seasoned sorcerer.

❀ ❀ ❀

In Niger, sorcerers are usually solitary figures. They usually live at the edge of town and serve as physical intermediaries between the calm tranquility of the village and the chaotic danger of the bush. Situated at the edge of reality, the sorcerer is utterly alone. Although sorcerers are, like anyone else, members of families and networks of friends, these associates cannot help them to confront the underside of the world. Sorcerers are the solitary spiritual guardians of their communities. Through ritual incantations and offerings, they attempt to balance the disruptive forces of the bush, which, in turn, creates harmony in the world. In a harmonious context, sorcerers attempt to develop their vision. They throw cowry shells to see bits of the past, present, and future. The shells chart a course on which sorcerers are eventually able to cut through life's haze and see things clearly. After years of concentrated effort the capacity to see things more clearly than others develops into a seasoned humility. Seasoned sorcerers come to understand how they are a relatively small part of a great tradition—a trickle in the flow of history. Accordingly, they realize that the knowledge they have acquired is borrowed and that their responsibility is to refine what they have learned and pass it on to the next generation. Ideally, this humility enables them to be more comfortable in their skins and gives them the courage to confront the world with a degree of strength and dignity; it can enable them to live well in the world.

Like Songhay sorcerers, cancer patients are also solitary figures. The disease makes you the intermediary between the relative tranquility of family life and the absolute disruption of illness. You live at the edge of the village of the sick. You can see your friends and family in the village of the healthy. Although you can visit them frequently, your place is elsewhere. Your life on the edge makes you a lonely figure in the world. Like the Songhay sorcerer, you, too, can use ritual, both spiritual and pragmatic, to establish harmony in your world. Like the Songhay sorcerer, you, too, can try to see things clearly and develop a strong-willed humility. Like the sorcerer, you can realize that time on earth is borrowed and must be eventually paid back. This realization can make you more comfortable with yourself and give you the courage to confront the existential imponderables of being diagnosed with and treated for cancer.

CHAPTER THREE

Treatment

On the day of my first chemotherapy treatment I sat in one of the medical recliners in The Cancer Center's infusion room and pondered my uncertain future. Waiting to begin this unexpected, uncertain, and painful part of my life, I realized that the *genji how*, which I had recited to calm myself, had not completely dissipated my fear of chemotherapy. Before I had excessively pondered my fate, Jennifer, my oncology nurse, returned. She stood next to the wooden barrier that divided the room into alcoves. She arranged an array of plastic tubes, needles, and several bulging plastic bags, the repository of anticancer drugs. She wrote notes and looked at the table next to my recliner.

"I see you came well prepared," she said cheerfully. "What's all that stuff?" she asked as she looked at my *bogolanfini* cloth, cassette recorder, cassettes, and energy bars.

"If I'm going to be here for five hours," I said, "I want to be as comfortable as possible. The cloth is a slice of home. The jazz tapes will hopefully take me away to a more peaceful place."

"Good idea." Infusion needle in hand, she sat down on a swivel chair and pushed herself in front of me. "Where's your brother?" she asked.

"He had to make some phone calls."

She looked at my hands. "Which one?"

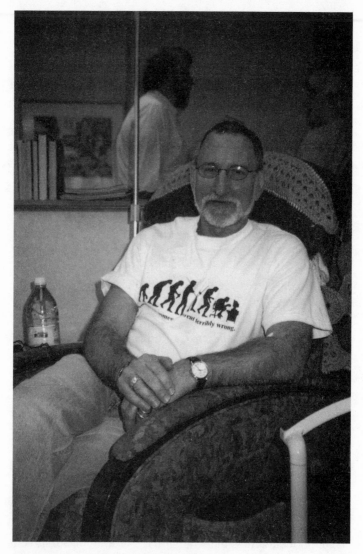

The author in the infusion room of The Cancer Center (2001).
Photo: Jasmin Tahmaseb McConatha

"Left," I said, not telling her that among the Songhay, the left hand is the seat of power. Sorcerers wear their power objects—rings and bracelets—on the left side of the body.

She took hold of my left hand and tapped my veins, looking for a suitable candidate. "Are you okay?"

"Yes," I said, lying.

"If you need anything, just let me know. We'll do this step by step, and I'll be with you."

I managed a weak smile and took a deep breath.

Jennifer found a good vein and pierced it with the infusion needle. Two small tubes were attached to it. Cytoxan and Rituxan would be dripped into my bloodsteam through the larger of the two tubes. Jennifer would inject a smaller dose of the powerful vincristine into the smaller tube, the top of which was covered by taut rubber—the site of the injection. She put a stopper in the larger tube. "We're just about ready." She gave me four steroid tablets. "Take these," she said. "They prevent nausea."

She then handed me four sheets of paper that described the potential side effects of the drugs that would soon be infused into my body. The first document, produced by a company that manufactured anticancer drugs, discussed chemotherapy's usual side effects—hair loss, mouth sores, nausea, and infection. It also mentioned what you could do to minimize side effects. There was little that could be done, according to the document, to prevent hair loss. The best strategy, which I followed one day prior to my initial treatment session, was to get a buzz cut to reduce the psychological shock of being suddenly bald. Cancer patients were also advised to use mild shampoos, soft hairbrushes, and the low heat setting on hair dryers. Mouth sores, tender gums, and sore throat, which usually occurred seven to fourteen days after the beginning of treatment, was yet another side effect of chemotherapy. The anticancer drugs not only kill malignant cells, but also destroy mucosal cells, which leads to mucositis. Here the document recommends a bland, soft diet. You wash down this soft bland food with plenty of fluids and make sure to frequently brush your teeth with mild toothpaste and a soft brush. Nausea is perhaps the most widely known side effect of chemotherapy. When chemotherapy drugs kill healthy cells, substances that make you sick to your stomach are released into the blood. Drugs and dietary adjustment, according to the document, can minimize nausea. The most serious chemotherapy side effect is infection. Chemotherapy drugs reduce the number of infection-fighting white blood cells. Accordingly, chemotherapy patients are highly prone to a variety of infections. The document writers recommend daily temperature taking, frequent hand washing, daily baths or showers, the use of electric razors, and proper food handling. They also suggest that you avoid crowds, immunization shots, fever-reducing aspirin, and the squeezing of pimples.

After reading the first document, I looked up at Jennifer, who continued to make notations on my chart. "Pretty bleak picture," I said. "How do you avoid crowds?"

"It's usually not as bad as they say," she said. "Each person reacts differently. Side effects also depend upon the drug combination you get."

"Am I going to lose my hair?"

"It's good you got a buzz cut," she said, "you know, to prepare people. If you're getting Cytoxan, your hair should be gone in about two weeks."

I appreciated her candor. "Do you think a gold or silver earring would look good on my ear?"

She smiled. "Go for the gold."

"Left or right ear?"

"Left." She nodded. "Paul, it's real good to maintain a sense of humor, if you can." She paused a moment. "Before we go on, you need to read the other sheets and then sign a release form."

I looked at the other documents, prepared by staff at The Cancer Center, which described the side effects of the drugs I would be getting. Cytoxan causes bone marrow suppression, which decreases white blood cells as well as platelets. White blood cells fight infection; platelets clot the blood. Cytoxan could cause fever, chills, red skin sores, severe cough, and a sore throat. It could also increase bruising and produce blood in the urine or stool and make your gums or nose bleed. In addition, it could provoke nausea, hair loss, and irritation of the bladder.

"Nasty stuff," I observed.

"You really need to drink as much water as possible. You don't want that stuff hanging around your bladder."

I moved on to vincristine, which, like Cytoxan, reduced your white cells and platelets. It also suppressed red blood cells, a factor that could bring on fatigue. Vincristine could also cause constipation and hair loss. If it leaked out from the vein, it could ulcerate the surrounding soft tissue. Its most serious side effect, though, was neurological, for it could cause tingling, numbness, and cramping in the extremities. The neurological effects, moreover, were cumulative. In time, vincristine could produce peripheral neuropathy, the loss of sensation in the feet and hands. In the most severe cases, neuropathy might make it difficult to walk or weaken your hand grasp. Other side effects include shortness of breath, double vision, and severe jaw, arm, back, or leg pain. Jennifer noticed my furrowed brow. "You only get a small dose of it," she said reassuringly.

I moved on to prednisone, a widely prescribed anti-inflammatory drug that also suppresses white-blood-cell counts and shrinks tumors. Massive doses of this steroid could produce multiple side effects that include nausea, anorexia, increased appetite, rash, acne, poor wound healing, insomnia, muscle weakness, euphoria, psychosis, depression, headache, dizziness, seizures, fluid retention, hypertension, blood clots, increased blood sugar, osteoporosis and back pain, herpes, and fungal infections. The dose that I'd be taking, of course, made me a prime candidate for one or more of these charming conditions.

I shook my head.

"Here's the thing with chemotherapy," Jennifer said. "The trick is to try to live with the side effects. If you can make adjustments, your life can remain kind of normal." She looked at the Rituxan pamphlet she had given me. "Well, at least one of the drugs you're getting has limited side effects."

Unlike the chemotherapy drugs and steroids, Rituxan, the antibody that attaches to a surface protein on lymphoma cells, seemed to have limited side effects. Most of the usually mild side effects occurred during the first infusion, which nurses administer gradually. These include fever, chills, headache, and nausea.

Nowhere in the documents did it say: "Reading these documents may produce nausea." The story of side effects, though, made me sick to my stomach. "I've read everything. It's a scary scenario," I said.

"It's tough," Jennifer said. "You'll need to be patient. Let's hope that the treatments will get you into a very long remission." She handed me the release form, which I signed.

In the back of my mind, I heard Adamu Jenitongo's voice saying, "The world is patience. The world is patience." Good advice, I thought, but difficult to heed when you're feeling nauseous.

"Are you ready?" Jennifer asked.

I nodded.

She positioned the IV bag on the metallic IV tree and then connected the IV line to the tube attached to the infusion needle. She then started a flow of saline into my bloodsteam. It felt cool as it flowed through my arm.

"Is it supposed to feel cool?" I asked.

"That's good," she said. "If it feels hot or itchy, let me know. That's not good."

"Okay."

She picked up a small syringe filled with yellow fluid. "This is vincristine. I'm going to slowly inject it into this small tube," she explained, referring to the small, rubber-sealed tube near my wrist.

I immediately imagined it leaking from the vein. How would it feel to have this drug burn soft tissue and skin?

She injected the needle into the rubber end of the tube and slowly pushed the yellow fluid into the IV line and my bloodstream. I averted my eyes for what was an interminable moment.

"All finished," she said. "You okay?"

I nodded again.

She then took a large fat syringe filled with Cytoxan and injected 1,750 milligrams of it through a rubber injection site on the IV bag and adjusted the IV flow meter. "Let me know if you need anything," she said. "You'll probably get a metallic taste in your mouth. Suck on some hard candy and drink plenty of water."

She returned to the nurse's station to monitor other patients. Heeding the warning about the negative effects of Cytoxan, I began to take sips from one of two large bottles of mineral water. As I felt the cool surge of Cytoxan moving through my body, my brother returned.

"How's it going?" he asked somewhat nervously.

How are you supposed to talk to a person undergoing his or her first chemotherapy treatment? I wondered. How are you supposed to talk to someone who, despite an attempted front of confidence and good humor, is afraid of dying a painful death? As normally as possible, I said to myself.

"It could be worse," I replied.

He sat down next to me and we talked at length about family and the excellent soccer play of his younger daughter, Lauren. We talked about our mother, who lived in Florida, and discussed our father, who had died the year before. Mitch also talked about various fund-raising campaigns he had organized for the Christopher Reeve Foundation. We told stories about our cousins, aunts, and uncles.

"How do you feel?" Mitch asked.

I looked up at the nearly depleted bag. "Aside from the metallic taste in my mouth, I don't feel too bad." I took another drink of water. "My arms feel heavy." I carefully pushed myself out of the recliner. "I have to pee." Pushing the IV tree along the floor, I slowly made my way to the bathroom and maneuvered the IV line so that I could relieve myself—no easy task. My mission completed, I shuffled back to the infusion room.

Shortly after my return to the recliner, the Cytoxan bag was empty. Jennifer, who moved like a gentle breeze in her white slacks and blue print smock, glided back to me. She removed the spent bag of Cytoxan and positioned two smaller bags on the tree.

"What are those?"

"To prep you for the Rituxan you get Benadryl followed by Tagamet." She handed me three tablets of Tylenol. "Take these."

I swallowed the tablets.

"Are you ready for the Benadryl?"

I nodded.

"It'll make you drowsy. Lots of people fall asleep."

"For that," I asserted, "I know I'm ready!"

In short order, I felt sleepy. I tried unsuccessfully to continue my conversation with Mitch. A state of blissful incoherence overcame me. Mitch smiled at my attempts to talk.

"I'm slurring my words."

"You might say that." He chuckled. "Maybe you should put on your jazz tapes," he suggested. "I'll read a little and then go and make some more phone calls."

"Sure," I said, as the sounds of John Coltrane's saxophone entered my ears. I closed my eyes and imagined myself sitting on a Nigerien sand dune as the sun set over the Niger River.

After an uncertain amount of time Jennifer tapped my wrist. "How are you, Paul?"

I opened my eyes. "Oh, I'm out there," I said. "This is the best part of chemotherapy, right?"

"It's more agreeable than the other stuff," she admitted. "I'm going to start the Rituxan. We give it very slowly. You need to tell me if you get chills, feel hot, or get short of breath."

I nodded.

She opened the flow of Rituxan into my bloodstream. From within a Benadryl haze, I wondered if I'd get chills or a fever from the antibodies, cloned from mice, which were flowing into my body. I looked up and watched the slow drip of clear fluid moving through the IV line. I dozed off and imagined a scene from Paul Bowles's *The Sheltering Sky*. In the scene, Port Moresby, the protagonist, is dying of typhoid fever in some forgotten corner of the Sahara. The high fever, which eventually kills him, provokes blood red hallucinations and chilling screams.

Jennifer's presence, which I somehow sensed, freed me from the daydream and its imagery.

"You okay?"

"I'm better off awake," I said. "Bad dreams."

"The effects of the Benadryl are probably starting to wear off," she stated. "Since you're okay, I'll increase the flow so that we can get out of here."

After an hour of Rituxan, only one-quarter of the prescribed dose had emptied into my body. I looked up at the bag. "How much longer?"

"Probably another two hours."

I put in another tape and closed my eyes, but did not fall asleep. Having already spent four hours at The Cancer Center, I felt more weary than sleepy.

I tried to read the book I had brought, an anthropological study of spirit possession in Niger, but found the prose and the topic far too complex for my state of mind. I passed the time listening to music and observing other patients. Although the infusion room had been designed to promote conversation—and solidarity among cancer patients—patients daydreamed, slept, read, or talked to family members. Few of them conversed with one another.

Long after everyone else had finished and gone home, the IV had finally emptied itself into my body. Jennifer detached me from the IV line, made a few more notations on my chart, and closed my file. "Are you okay?"

I felt no pain and was grateful to be free of nausea. "Not too bad," I admitted.

"Good," she said. "If you have any problems, give us a call, and make sure to drink plenty of water."

"Believe me, I won't forget."

She handed me my file. "Take that to the front desk. They'll schedule your next treatment session—"

"In three weeks," I said, finishing her sentence for her as I struggled to get out of my chair. Although I had not experienced any pain, I felt as if my body had been flooded with fluids. My arms felt heavy and immobile; my legs felt like water-soaked tree trunks. My head felt fuzzy. Followed by Mitch, I walked toward the empty waiting room, which in my weary state, looked like one of Monet's fuzzy impressionist paintings. Did the hazy reality of impressionism, I wondered, emerge from an artist's confrontation with perception-altering pain? The receptionist signed me up for my next session—a five-hour reservation for one of the medical recliners in the infusion room.

"Don't you ever leave here?" I asked her.

"We don't leave until the last patient leaves." Her tone was cheerful, considering that it was after 6:00 P.M. on a Friday.

"I'm sorry," I said.

"We're here to do what we can for you, Paul."

She gave me a prescription for prednisone and an order form for blood work. "If you get a fever or rash, just call. We'll look after you."

"Thank you."

Mitch and I walked out into the gray dusk light. A cool breeze brushed my face. I opened the car door and I tried to squeeze my heavy body into the car seat. We started our trip back to my apartment. Much like our trip to The Cancer Center earlier in the day, we made small talk—observations about the weather or the news. Mitch then asked me how I felt.

"A little bit tired, but otherwise okay," I said. I began to wonder how I'd be able to endure at least eight months of chemotherapy treatment, the usual time frame of initial chemotherapy for NHL. I finally dozed off and awoke as we pulled into the driveway of my apartment building.

Miriam had volunteered to take me for my first treatment. When I decided to go with my brother, she had offered to come over and cook a light meal. When we walked into my apartment the soothing aroma of rice and chicken kebabs welcomed us. Surprisingly, the aroma of good food made me hungry. Miriam handed Mitch a beer and gave me a bottle of mineral water.

"I'm actually hungry," I said.

"That must be a good sign," Miriam said.

Mitch decided to skip dinner and head home. "If you need anything," he said hastily, "just let me know."

I was sure he was eager to return to his family and a sense of normality. I did not blame him. I appreciated his efforts to be there for me on that difficult day.

What the social psychologists say about social support, I thought at that moment, is largely true.[1] My brother's willingness to accompany me to my first treatment had meant a lot to me. I had appreciated the phone calls and cards I had received from family members after the diagnosis. Their expressions of concern made me feel better. Why is it, I wondered, that bad news and suffering often propel distant family members into proximity? As I prepared for bed that night, though, I realized yet again that cancer patients—me, in this instance—must live alone with a disease that their own bodies had produced. It was, I realized, an exclusive relationship with oneself, a relationship that separated us even more from the people in our lives, making us more alone in the world.

❁ ❁ ❁

That night I fell into a fitful sleep. My body felt heavy and numb. I dreamed of Adamu Jenitongo. We had been transported back to the early part of the twentieth century. In his early years my mentor walked hundreds of kilometers across West Africa to perform circumcisions. In the dream, I served as his assistant. We traveled to one elaborately built village in the West African grasslands. The mud-brick, straw-roofed houses seemed to swirl like a cluster of stars from the village center. Just beyond the edge of the village swirl, we came upon a large group of men and boys. They greeted us. My teacher took out his circumcising knives and a piece of slate he used to sharpen the blades.

"Make these sharp," he said to me as he gave me the instruments. "They must be very sharp."

I began to sharpen the knives, which were, in fact, scalpels.

Adamu Jenitongo then produced some seeds and green powder. After each circumcision, he'd chew on a seed and spit on the wound to dull the pain. He'd then moisten the powder into healing paste that would be applied to the wound.

Soon fathers accompanied their sons to the site of circumcision. For each circumcision, Adamu Jenitongo recited a special incantation that set the world straight. He then performed the rite for every uncircumcised boy in the village. In one afternoon, he circumcised more than fifty boys. In the evening, village elders slaughtered a cow and roasted its meat in our honor. We ate with abandon. As their sons recuperated, the village elders drank millet beer, talked, joked, and celebrated an important milestone.

The next morning we left for the next village. Walking along a narrow path that cut through tall elephant grass, we suddenly heard a deep growl. As we turned a bend on the path, we came upon an adult female lion. We froze in our tracks. I trembled with fear. Adamu Jenitongo remained calm.

"Lion, we come here with respect. We are both on the path," he stated calmly.

The lion growled.

Adamu Jenitongo turned to me. "As with everything else, you stand your ground against lions. We both live in the world. We are both on the path. Gather your strength and stand your ground."

The standoff lasted for several moments. Finally, the lion lost interest and wandered off into the elephant grass.

"I guess we won that battle," I said, greatly relieved.

"No, we didn't," Adamu Jenitongo said. "Lions always return. What's important is that you faced the lion and stood your ground."

I awoke from the dream with reinforced determination. Like my mentor and teacher, I told myself, I'd try to face my new ordeal—cancer—with respect. I rolled out of bed. The heaviness left in the wake of the chemotherapy infusion remained, making me stiff and sluggish. Although I wanted to go back to bed, I forced myself to stand on an Oriental rug positioned at the foot of my bed. Slowly and with a lot of effort, I performed a series of yoga stretches, a routine I had learned twenty years earlier. I did breathing exercises and meditated for five minutes.

Miriam came by with some fresh bread and feta cheese. She made a pot of tea. The food and tea settled my stomach and tasted surprisingly good. I had one more morning task: to take nine twenty-milligram tablets of bitter-tasting prednisone. Soon I felt remarkably better. The heaviness in my limbs slipped away. My hunger increased. I even felt up to taking a short walk.

"Hang in there," Miriam said. "It's really important to do as much as possible without exhausting yourself—go to dinner, teach, write, travel."

"I agree," I said.

"If you feel up to it, we can go around the corner this evening to have dinner at that small Italian place."

After Miriam had left for work, I tried to read and write a little, but couldn't concentrate. The effects of prednisone filled me with what seemed boundless nervous energy. For hours, I sat at my computer desk and searched the Internet for cancer-related links. I subscribed to a variety of newsletters that would send me the latest cancer news—even news about the molecular structure and treatment of NHL. I also searched sites for an image of the small-cleaved follicular lymphoma cell. I had seen the CAT-scan image of my abdominal tumor, but wanted to visualize the cells that constituted it. My plan was to visualize the tumor cells and then to imagine them being slowly destroyed. I wanted to "see" antibodies attaching themselves to antigens (proteins) on lymphoma cells. This event would trigger macrophage action. Macrophages, the Pac-Men of the cellular world, would then gobble up these marked-for-death lymphoma cells. I wanted to see hundreds of macrophages streaking like meteorites to the tumor site. I wanted to envision the tumor slowly but inexorably shrinking after each sortie of macrophages. I wanted to be an active participant in this struggle with what my own body had produced. I wanted to regain a measure of control over my own bodily processes.

Several hours passed by in a flash. Friends called to check on me, but mostly I lost myself in my tasks, a phenomenon psychologists call "flow," which is considered therapeutic. After a long period of "flow," I stretched my back and stood up. My heart beat wildly and I felt a slight dizziness. Deciding I needed some fresh air, I went outside. I wanted to stroll along the Brandywine River, which is a short walk from my apartment. At first, I walked somewhat briskly without incident. After about ten minutes my legs felt heavy and rubbery and my head started to spin. I quickly went back home and lay down for one hour. As a chemotherapy patient, I realized, I may be able to write, lecture, even travel a bit, but there would certainly be limits and bad as well as good days. I had a lot of adjusting to do.

As the last rays of the sun stretched across my living room, I decided to go out that evening. I phoned Miriam and arranged to have dinner at seven.

After we were seated at the restaurant, Miriam ordered a glass of white wine. I asked for a glass of mineral water. The lights had been dimmed. Could anyone guess, I wondered, that I had had a chemotherapy treatment the previous day? How many other people sitting in restaurants at that very moment shared my situation?

Miriam raised her glass. "To you, Paul. Who would have thought that you'd be having dinner out one day after your first treatment? Bravo!"

We clinked our glasses. Over my left shoulder, I felt the presence of Adamu Jenitongo and smiled.

❀ ❀ ❀

The ongoing presence of my mentor did not surprise me. To be sure, he was an important person in my life and my memories of him have remained strong. The sense of his presence, though, was more than a memory. Among many peoples of the world, the dead, as ancestors, play important and active roles in the present. People make offerings to them to ensure a productive hunt or an abundant harvest.[2] The Songhay people are no exception to this pattern, especially so if you are connected to a family of sorcerers. In some respects, sorcerers like Adamu Jenitongo defy death itself.[3] Family members feel their presence long after their deaths. Presence is felt in what are called sorcerer dreams, through which master sorcerers, though long dead, continue the education of their apprentices. These dreams can provide both explicit and metaphorical lessons. There are circumstances in which apprentices hear their master's voice—especially at pivotal moments in their lives. Sometimes apprentices actually feel the presence of their mentors, a sensation that can provide deep comfort during intensely stressful moments. The connection between master and apprentice is materially reinforced. Among the Songhay, many people believe that the sorcerer's immaterial essence—his or her spirit—can live in material objects like stones, rings, bracelets, and iron staffs. The power of the master's spirit can lay dormant for years until the danger of serious illness, for example, ignites its force. If you possess these objects you are, in fact, continuously connected to your mentor.[4]

❊ ❊ ❊

The reassuring spirit presence of Adamu Jenitongo did not free me from the emergence of searing pain, which began three days after my first chemotherapy treatment. Over the weekend, I had felt tired, but otherwise okay. My appetite remained strong. No painful mouth sores had appeared on my lip or tongue. Thankfully, my hair hadn't fallen out. Infection hadn't raised my body temperature. Even though I had read that the onset of chemotherapy's side effects is gradual, I had braced myself to deal with the pain and disruption of cancer treatment. I tried to dismiss my treatment—and even cancer—as no big deal. My ill-conceived arrogance lasted only two days. Waking up on the third day of being a chemotherapy patient, my head hurt, my neck ached, and my shoulders throbbed. The small of my back felt as if someone was slowly tightening a screw into a bone socket; each turn fired a flame of pain through my legs.

Slowly I rolled out of bed and walked to the bathroom to take some Tylenol, the painkiller of choice for chemotherapy patients. You don't want to take any painkiller with ibuprofen, my nurses told me, because it further affects platelets already depleted by chemotherapy drugs. Fortified with Tylenol and carrying my vial of prednisone, I slowly made my way down the long hallway of my apartment, walked across the living room, and continued through the dining room to the galley kitchen.

The effort was enormous. Overnight the apartment seemed to have expanded to ten times its original size. In the kitchen I found a bottle of cold water. Standing at the counter, I swallowed my nine prednisone tablets. I hoped that the prednisone would provide jolts of energy that would dissipate the aches and pains. It didn't. After eating a bowl of usually comforting oatmeal, I lay down on the living room sofa. How was I supposed to go to work? To get to work, I'd have to shower, get dressed, stuff myself in my low-riding Saturn, drive fifteen miles along winding roads, and park the car in the distant student-faculty lot. Once parked, I'd still have to walk a half mile to my building on campus and climb four flights of stairs to my office. Because anthropologists are usually associated with old things, universities—and mine is no exception—often house anthropology departments in their oldest, most decrepit buildings. Once in my office, I'd have to hold office hours and talk with students. In the past, I hadn't given the slightest thought to these small tasks. Thinking about my difficulties, I remembered a conversation with an older neighbor who, despite having had recent heart bypass surgery, managed to not only drive his car, but load and unload his groceries.

"How do you do it?" I asked.

"I pace myself," he said, smiling. "That's all there is to it."

I now followed his advice, for I had to learn to live with cancer, but somehow not allow it to take over my life. And so, like thousands of other chemotherapy patients, I decided to go to work. I showered and dressed slowly and with deliberation. I drove to the university. I walked to my office building. I climbed the stairs one floor at a time and breathed a sigh of relief when I finally reached my office. I then took some Tylenol, drank lots of water, and tried to appear as "normal" as possible to students and colleagues.

My efforts appeared to be successful. The aches and pains didn't subside, but I got somewhat used them. After I told my colleagues about my lymphoma diagnosis, they arranged for a couch to be placed in my office. The couch afforded me a place where, when in need of rest, I could lay down for thirty minutes, a short but restorative interlude. Even so, I wondered how I would fare in the classroom. Jolted by the effects of chemotherapy drugs, could I talk enthusiastically about anthropology for seventy-five minutes? Should I tell my students that I had cancer? Following the wisdom of Adamu Jenitongo, I decided to be honest with them.

Three days after my first treatment, I walked into the classroom and faced forty-five students, some eager, some anxious, some bored. The subject that day was the origin of the state. What factors precipitated the change from egalitarian subsistence societies in which everyone did similar work and lived in similar circumstances to complex societies in which the work of the many provided for the wealth of the few? This lecture, one of my favorites, was usually one that captured the interest of my students.

I cleared my throat. My shoulders and back still ached from the treatment. "Good afternoon."

Several students muttered a greeting. Most of them stared at me as they waited for the lecture to begin.

"Before we get started, I want to say something." I paused a moment. "In the coming weeks, my appearance might change. I may start looking like Mr. Clean." I took a deep breath. "I've been diagnosed with cancer and last Friday I had my first chemotherapy treatment. I hope to continue teaching," I continued slowly, "but I thought I should let you know." I paused and looked at my students and wondered if any of them had been touched by cancer. I smiled. "I've got two questions. When I'm completely bald, I'd like to get an earring. Which ear should I get pierced? And should the earring be silver or gold?"

They smiled. One female student raised her hand. "Get the gold and put it on the left ear."

On that note I began my lecture. Pain quickly took a backseat to the origin of the state.

After the lecture several students came up to express their concern as well as their opinions on the kind of earring I should order.

"It's good you told us, Dr. Stoller," one student said. "We think professors are so different. This makes you seem more like us."

Several other students voiced similar sentiments, all of which made my spirits soar.

⌘   ⌘   ⌘

The Songhay way had once again steered me in the right direction. When you are diagnosed with cancer, as I have said, you enter a new world, which in mainstream American culture, following the wisdom of Susan Sontag, is a dark, fearful domain of pain and suffering. It is a place where most people don't want to go. It is a place most people don't want to talk about. These stigmatic realities create a quandary. Whom should you tell about your cancer? Once you've decided whom you should tell, how do you talk about it to them? And once people know that you have cancer, how often and when should you discuss it with them? There are, of course, no easy answers to these questions. It's relatively easy to tell people in your circle of family and close friends, who will react, if my experience is any indication, with great variation. How you approach your acquaintances and colleagues is another matter. In some cases, I wish that I hadn't told some of my associates that I was a cancer patient, for it prompted distance and avoidance, which is understandable but sad. What is more important, following the wisdom of Songhay teachings, is to be comfortable with your situation, which in Songhay culture means that you try to see things clearly and are correct with yourself. This stance enables you to accept your vulnerability, a state that opens your being to other people, which in turn helps to promote a degree of quiet dignity to which most people respond positively.

In some circumstances, though, it is almost impossible to be comfortable. As I shoved more and more prednisone into my body, my heart, beating ever more rapidly, seemed to migrate to my throat. No amount of food could satisfy my hunger. I slept fitfully and grew increasingly irritable with friends and family. Although my aches and pains increased cumulatively, I tried to maintain my schedule. I got up early, did yoga stretches, meditated, made offerings upon my altar, and recited Songhay incantations. After several days the pain and anxiety reached a climax and then slowly, like rising fog, dissipated. Ten days into the three-week treatment cycle, my energy returned. Sleep came more easily. My appetite stabilized. My mood improved. On those good days I went to the gym to work out. Even though a short twenty-minute workout was exhausting, the accomplishment encouraged me.

Doing anthropological fieldwork had always been among the most rewarding aspects of my career, a part of my life I was unwilling to give up. On the good days following chemotherapy treatments, I tried to squeeze in some fieldwork in New York City. On my first visit there after having been diagnosed, my West African friends at the Malcolm Shabazz Harlem Market received me with warmth.

After hugging me, Issifi Mayaki, a cloth trader, showed me into his little shop. We exchanged family news and talked about the local and world economy.

"Paul," Issifi said, "you look pale. Are you okay?"

"No," I answered. "I'm afraid I've got cancer. I've started chemotherapy."

Issifi grimaced and shook his head. "Why is it that misfortune strikes good people and steers away from thieves and good-for-nothings?" He paused. "What do the doctors say?"

"They say that the cancer I have can be managed for a long time. They say I'll need eight months to a year of chemotherapy."

"My wife had breast cancer. When she got diagnosed two years ago and had surgery and chemotherapy, she kept saying, 'I'm gonna die; I'm gonna die.' I told her to be patient. I told her that my father would recite the Alfatia [the Muslim prayer for protection] for her. She's doing well now and the cancer has not come back."

"Would you recite the Alfatia for me?"

"I will do it when I next go to pray," he said. "I will also talk to my father in Abidjan and ask him to recite it for you."

Issifi hugged me again. "You are going be okay. I know it." He smiled. "You'll be in my thoughts. Go and see the others."

I walked to Boubé Mounkaila's shop, and we shook hands and exchanged greetings. We had known one another for almost ten years. I told him about my cancer.

Boubé put his arm around my shoulder. "Sit down. Sit."

"Your body may feel weak," he said when I had seated myself, "but I know that your spirit is strong. You will come out of this. I know it."

After visiting several other traders, I left the market with a feeling of great gratitude. How wonderful, I thought, to know firsthand the deep humanity of my West African trader friends. They accepted my cancerous state directly and positively.

As I approached the end of the first three-week cycle of chemotherapy, I realized what my near future would entail. As the chemotherapy agents destroyed healthy as well as malignant cells during the first half of the three-week cycle, my body would throb, especially in the neck, shoulders, and back. In time, my throat would burn. I might get sores on my tongue, cheeks, and lips. Periodic fevers would make me sweat. Rashes might spread over my body. And just as my body had cleansed itself of the poisons that precipitated this misery, I'd once again have to drag myself to The Cancer Center. If my blood work produced acceptable results, I'd be hooked up for another treatment and another three-week cycle of side effects. How many of these cycles would I face: eight, twelve, sixteen?

The prospect of a long period of chemotherapy considerably darkened my horizons. And yet I tried to maintain my spirits. I still had my hair, and much of my energy. I hoped that I could use the wisdom of Songhay sorcery, embodied in the memory and image of Adamu Jenitongo, to chart a good path through the village of the sick. Would I emerge from chemotherapy unscathed? I now knew that my life would never return to "normal." Cancer and chemotherapy treatments would leave their mark on me.

"You can stop the chemotherapy anytime you want," one of my friends asserted after hearing vivid descriptions of the side effects.

"Yes," I said, "but what's the alternative?"

❀ ❀ ❀

The agonizingly slow and indecisive process of diagnosis had forced me to confront the past, present, and future of my life. It was an exceedingly frustrating time. I had to wait for results, which were usually inconclusive, and then arrange for more diagnostic tests, which required preparation and some degree of grit. The world of diagnosis is nothing less than a physical and emotional whirlwind that completely disrupts your life.

Treatment is an altogether different matter. In treatment the world slows down. You must sit for hours as the chemotherapy drugs drip into your bloodstream. The drugs make your body ache. They make you tired. You have to pace yourself. They force you to be patient. Patience is the password into the village of the sick.

In contemporary society, patience, as I've indicated earlier in this book, is usually beside the point. Things in mainstream American culture are complex and ever changing. Most of us like quick car trips and fast computers and a pace of life that includes a multitude of activities.[5] I've also said that most Songhay people expect delays when they travel. In Niger, the pace of life is relatively slow, especially in the countryside, where most people have no electricity and running water. In the mornings you work. In the heat of the day, you move slowly and take a siesta. In the late afternoon, you work some more. In the evening you talk with your friends.

The pace of apprenticeship is also slow and deliberate. Sorcerers must be patient if they want to learn about plants, potions, and power. As already stated, many sorcerers among the Songhay must wait more than thirty years before their "paths" open. There are many Songhay proverbs that speak to the necessity of deliberate preparation.[6] Individuals who embark on a task before they are ready to do so, these proverbs suggest, invariably fail. In sorcery, lack of preparation can sometimes result in misfortune, sickness, and even death. I did not fully understand the importance of this primary element of Songhay culture until the power of cancer and the effect of chemotherapy drugs forced me to live life at a more deliberate pace. What was my alternative?

❋ ❋ ❋

After three cycles of chemotherapy, Joel Rubin sent me for a CAT scan. He wanted to see if the regimen of Cytoxan, vincristine, prednisone, and Rituxan was working. Once again I drank two containers of the unpleasant barium and asked Miriam to drive me to Community Radiology Services. We arrived at the appointed time.

I was a CAT-scan veteran. I knew how to prepare to be scanned. I knew several of the technicians. Still, when Bill, the nurse who would inject iodine into my vein, articulated the required litany of potential complications, I shuddered. "Don't worry, Paul," he said, "these things hardly ever occur."

I soon heard the whir and whine of the CAT scanner. The disembodied voice repeatedly instructed me to hold and let out my breath. Bill came in and pushed the iodine into my veins. I again feared that I would have an allergic reaction. Finally, Bill came back into the room.

"We're finished."

He disconnected me from the infusion line and I was left to face the rest of my day—giving a final exam in my seminar. Before leaving, I asked the receptionist how long it would take to get the results.

"Three or four days."

As any patient knows, it is difficult to be patient when you are awaiting the results of medical tests—results that sometimes may change the course of your life. In most circumstances, results are not released to impatient patients; rather, they are forwarded to the physician who ordered the test. In some cases, the physician will ask you to make an appointment so that she or he can discuss the results. In other cases, you are asked to call for results. In my case, I phoned the nurses at The Cancer Center. I received a recorded announcement: "You've reached the nurses. If you are calling with a problem, please leave your name and phone number. If you are calling for results, please leave your name and phone number, the kind of test you had, and the name of your physician. We will get back to you as soon as we possibly can." This system is probably the most efficient one for dealing with a glut of phone calls from worried patients, but it assumes that you have the time to sit and wait for a phone call or that you have a cell phone. In my case, I don't own a cell phone, but I often worked at home, which made it possible—not easy—to sit and wait. While waiting I jumped every time the phone rang. Finally you get the call.

"Paul, this is Mary from Dr. Rubin's office."

"Hi, Mary," I said, trying to sound calm. "Did you get the results of my CAT scan?"

"I'm sorry," she said, "but they haven't been sent over yet. Try calling us back in two days."

"What's taking so long?" I asked, the hint of desperation in my voice. "Is there something wrong?"

"No, no," she said. "It sometimes takes a bit longer for them to send us the reports. That's all."

"Okay," I said, "I'll call again."

"Just try to put it out of your mind," she suggested.

"Easier said than done," I said. "Thanks anyway. I'll be in touch."

Two days later, I phoned The Cancer Center again. Having pushed the button for the nurses, the circuitry connected me to the same phone message. Dutifully, I left my name, number, doctor's name, and test. Thirty minutes later, Doris phoned me with the results.

"Paul, we have good news for you," she said. "The report says that your tumor has been reduced by fifty percent, and that there is no other evidence of disease progression. It says that you've had an excellent response to treatment. Congratulations."

Relief flooded through me. The treatments seemed to be working. On my next visit to The Cancer Center, Joel Rubin gave me the radiology report, which I scanned to reassure myself of its existence. I told him about the various side effects I had experienced. He agreed to reduce my dosage of steroids, which would hopefully make me less anxious and enable me to sleep more. He reassured me that I was responding quite well to the chemotherapy drugs and sent me off for my next treatment.

The CAT-scan results made me cautiously optimistic. Prior to my introduction to the twisted and confusing paths of the village of the sick, such results would have thrilled me. They would have reinforced a deeply rooted sense of invincibility. Several cycles of chemotherapy and my reconnection to Songhay traditions, however, had reinforced a sense of humility. Considering the results from the vantage of a pragmatic worldview, I braced myself for at least four more cycles of chemotherapy. Although I knew that I would be a cancer patient for the rest of my life, I hoped to complete my treatment and go into remission. Even if remission lasted many years, my condition would have to be monitored. During regularly spaced screening tests, the oncological team might find that the NHL had returned, which would mean that I'd have to seek new treatments. One day I might have to undergo a bone marrow transplant or stem cell replacement—risky procedures, to say the least. As I stared at my shrinking tumor, I remembered Adamu Jenitongo's words: "Expend your energy on what's important."

When you look at your own tumor on an x-ray board, you think more about what's important. You think about how you can use limited amounts of energy to squeeze little pleasures from life. Before cancer came into my life, I took pleasure from writing, from cooking, drinking good wine, from traveling, and from spending time with my friends.

During cancer treatment, though, things change. With the help of several friends, especially Miriam, I altered my life to accommodate the routine of three-week cycles of chemotherapy, reserving the most strenuous activities for the second ten days of the cycle. During those times, I visited my small beach house, took long walks along the shore, and even managed to canoe and kayak through nearby canals and back bays. These simple activities restored a sense of normality to my life and gave me more pleasure than they had before my diagnosis and treatment.

As summer approached I made tentative plans to travel overseas. I usually spent some time in France during the summer. This summer I hoped to visit old friends there and then spend a few days working in England with Miriam. I proceeded with my plans and pledged to pace myself on the trip. After an exhausting flight to England, Miriam and I spent several days in London, where we worked in the archives and attended lectures at University College, London, and the London School of Economics. We also took in some sights. Every day, we walked the streets of London, visited museums, and searched for reasonable restaurants that served decent food. The pace exhausted me. My body felt like it was on fire. Even so, I slogged on. I found relief in afternoon naps and in several twenty-minute chair massages. Never have massages felt so good!

I managed to spend a few pleasurable days in Paris but felt weak and tired. Even though I love Paris, I was ready to return home. The trip had been wonderful but a bit mad. Even so, I had no regrets and would have done it again.

Thankfully, Miriam had frequent-flyer miles and was able to get a business-class upgrade for our return flight. The upgrade made the trip home much more manageable—bigger, more comfortable chairs, more palatable food, and best of all, fresher air. When I returned home, though, I needed several days of rest to regain my equilibrium.

When I returned to The Cancer Center one week later and had my blood analyzed, I discovered that my white and red counts were not normal.

"Would that account for my fatigue?" I asked Joel Rubin, who wanted to hear about my adventures in Europe. "Is it my blood counts?"

"Probably not. The counts are low, but not that low. We can still proceed with treatment."

"Then why am I so tired?"

Joel shrugged his shoulders. "From what you describe, you might have done too much."

I nodded. "I thought I was taking it easy. I did much less than I usually do in Europe."

"Chemotherapy can also have a cumulative effect. The side effects become more pronounced as we move along."

"I suppose that gives me something to look forward to," I said. "At least this is the eighth treatment. It could be the last one," I added hopefully.

"Might be," Joel said. "Usually it takes eight months to a year of chemotherapy to treat NHL. I'll write you another CAT-scan order. Go during the next two weeks, and we'll see what's going on."

We shook hands and I walked back to the infusion room.

"Are you back again?" said Jennifer when she saw me.

"I can't get enough of this place."

"We should be getting near the end of your treatments."

"I hope so. I'm getting a CAT scan to see. I might need additional treatments, but this could be the last one."

"Let's hope so," she said, looking at my chart. "Pick a chair and I'll be back with your medicines."

❈ ❈ ❈

My treatment-induced weariness prompted me to think about the weariness of Songhay sorcerers, who continually complained about sleepless nights during which they confronted spirits and fought witches. As I stated earlier, the person in Songhay culture consists of three fundamental elements: flesh, spirit, and life force. When witches make a person sick, they steal her or his spirit and hide it. If they consume the person's spirit, he or she dies. But there is more to the story. Many Songhay believe that the spirit, which is their immaterial essence, leaves the body at night. Dreams recount the spirit's nocturnal adventures. Like anyone else, sorcerers have dreams, but they learn how to control the movement and actions of their spirits.

From their beds, they direct their spirits to ask the advice of supernatural beings, compete for power with the spirits of other sorcerers, and search for and neutralize witches. When the sorcerer's spirit encounters a witch, an incantation is recited.

DJILLO

> Djillo is in the darkness. In the darkness it sees a rock. And the rock sees the evil witch's genitalia. The lights of the witch flash on and off. But when it [the witch] lifts its torch, it is worthless because now it will fall and fear will escape. Men will not fear you. Women will not fear you. You will not know your front side from your back side. The darkness will be uplifted.[7]

If the witch or competitor proves to be more powerful than the sorcerer, then his or her spirit is vanquished, which means that when it returns to the sorcerer's sleeping body, it will promote aches, pains, or sickness in the sorcerer's flesh. Even in sleep, sorcerers, the spiritual guardians of their villages, get little if any rest. Theirs is a weariness of great spiritual obligation.

I once asked a yawning Sorko Djibo Mounmouni, the man who taught me the Djillo incantation, how he could accept such a state of weariness.

"I have no choice," he said. "It is my burden."

Like Sorko Djibo, cancer patients have no choice. They have to confront their weariness and make the necessary accommodations. It is a humbling exercise.

❄ ❄ ❄

Several days after my appointment with Joel Rubin, I made another trip to Community Radiology Services. I felt less anxiety about being sucked into the all-seeing bowels of the CAT scanner. Bruce, my nurse, took me back to the dressing rooms. I put on a hospital gown and he put a needle in my arm and attached a plastic tube to it—the pathway for iodine contrast.

"I have to ask you some questions," he stated.

"I know. I'm a CAT-scan veteran." I answered the questions about latex, allergies, fasting, asthma, and listened as he related the potentially lethal consequences of iodine.

In short order I lay on my back, arms stretched out over my head, and obeyed the commands to breathe and hold my breath. Bruce came in to administer the iodine contrast. As he slowly pushed the fluid into my body, he tapped my vein. "We should be finished soon."

This time, I felt the slow spread of the iodine through my body. As I tasted metal in my mouth, my throat constricted. My pulse raced. Should I say something now or wait? I could still breathe easily, but didn't want Bruce to rush in unnecessarily and pump adrenaline into my body. Should I or shouldn't I sound an alarm? As the iodine spread through my abdomen, my intestines shuddered. Was I going to die inside this infernal machine? The constricted feeling, however, lasted only an interminable moment. I relaxed.

"Are you okay in there?"

"Yes."

Three days later I phoned the nurses at The Cancer Center to get the results. I left my information on the answering machine and began the process of waiting. After a half-hour, one of the nurses phoned me.

"This is Dorothy calling from The Cancer Center."

"Yes . . ."

"I'm afraid we haven't yet received the results of your CAT scan. Call us back in two more days. The results should be in by then."

Why can't such important results be ready on time? I wondered. Two days later I was once again anxiously waiting for the phone to ring. I received several "courtesy calls" and a wrong number. Finally, I got a call from Karen, another of the nurses at The Cancer Center.

"Paul, I've got the CAT-scan report." She paused.

"Yes?"

"It says that the four-centimeter mass is still there, but there's no evidence of disease progression."

"You mean that the tumor hasn't shrunk any more," I said, my heart sinking.

"That's right."

"Then the treatments are no longer working," I stated flatly.

"Sometimes tumors don't disappear entirely," she said. "They become scar tissue. That's probably what's going on with you."

"But the last time, it shrank by fifty percent. I thought it would have just about disappeared by now."

"Don't be disheartened, Paul. According to this report, you're doing well."

"If you say so," I said, unconvinced.

Several days later, I took the latest CAT-scan images to an appointment with Joel Rubin. As I sat confined in the grim examination room, I pondered my fate. After the initial success of my treatment, I had redoubled my efforts to use alternative medicine to relieve side effects and reduce the size of my tumor. I received reflexology treatments, which energized me and offset the harsh effects of the chemo. Every Thursday and Sunday, I recited Songhay incantations and made offerings to the Songhay spirits. Every morning, I did yoga stretches. When I meditated, I envisioned macrophages destroying lymphoma cells. Each sortie reduced the tumor's size. Then I'd inhale deeply and envision dead lymphoma cells passing harmlessly out of my nostrils into the air. I had expected better results.

Joel came in and opened my chart. "How have you been?"

"The CAT-scan report disappointed me."

"You're at least in partial remission. You might be in complete remission," he asserted. He glanced at the large envelope on my lap. "Let's take a look at the film."

I followed him to the meeting room and watched as he put my insides on the backlit display case. He showed me what looked like identical images of the tumor—one taken in May, the other developed in August.

"There's not a lot of change," I said.

"Do you have a minute?"

"Of course."

"I want to run these over to the hospital and have my radiologist friend look at this film. You can wait in my office if you'd like."

Fifteen minutes later, Joel returned. "Good news," he said. "My friend says that the tumor looks much better now than it did in May. It's probably all scar tissue, but there could be traces of residual disease."

"You mean that most of the lymphoma cells are dead and gone, but there could be a few stragglers."

"That's right, especially in the center of the mass."

"What does that mean?"

"It means that we need another scan. I'm going to order a PET scan for you. This scan measures metabolic activity. They give you a radioactive tracer in a glucose solution, and the scan picks up activity of quickly dividing cells."

"Cancer cells."

"That's right. If there are any remaining lymphoma cells in the residual mass, the PET scan will pick it up."

"Sounds like a good idea."

Joel handed the file to me. "Take that up front and they'll give you the PET scan information. This is a new technology. Only two places in this entire region offer PET scans. Once you've had the scan we should know if you're in remission."

I took my file, brought it to the front desk, and received information on positron emission tomography. Thus armed, I readied myself for yet another adventure in the world of medicine.

❀ ❀ ❀

PET-scan technology is both new and expensive, which meant that at the time of my treatment only two medical facilities in the entire Philadelphia region offered these cutting-edge imaging services: Springfield Hospital in suburban Delaware County, Pennsylvania, and the University of Pennsylvania Hospital—a nationally designated cancer care center. Getting scheduled for a PET scan at the University of Pennsylvania is no easy task. You must phone early and pray that a human being will answer the phone. I had no such providential luck. I left my name and waited to be contacted. After two days, I decided to try Springfield Hospital and spoke to someone straightaway and scheduled my PET scan.

PET-scan imaging represents a significant advance in body imaging. When radiologists read a CAT scan, an MRI, an ultrasound, or an x-ray image, they look for differences in internal structure and anatomy to detect abnormal tissues, which in my case would be lymphoma cells. Radiologists analyzing PET-scan images look for differences in metabolic activity in tissues. Once the patient is injected with a radioactive solution, the PET scan can image the body's metabolic activity. Metabolic activity in cancerous tissues is more rapid than it would be in normal tissues and shows up as a dark spot. These dark spots can pinpoint cancerous activity too small to be detected by other imaging technologies.

Because each PET-scan study costs more than six thousand dollars, the hospitals that provide them require the patient to move through a series of "fail-safes" before she or he can qualify for the procedure. You need to have the "right" condition. PET scans are usually approved for lung cancer staging, melanoma, lymphoma, recurrent colon cancer, and solitary lung nodules. If you have such a condition, you then need a written note of pre-certification. Considering the "consequences" of the PET-scan results, clearing these bureaucratic hurdles is no easy psychological task. When I went through the ordeal, I remembered to breathe deeply. I also thought of Adamu Jenitongo urging me to be patient. Those physical and mental exercises made this stressful task a bit easier to bear.

My experience with this new technology started on a hot hazy day in August. Miriam, who had become my chauffeur and source of support during these stressful scans, drove me to Springfield Hospital, which is located on a manicured medical campus not far from the bucolic suburban enclave of Swarthmore, Pennsylvania. We parked in a designated spot and walked into the hospital's spacious, sparsely furnished reception hall. Tall windows ensured a flood of natural light. The place seemed deserted.

"There's hardly anyone here," I said to Miriam. "I hope that's not an indication of the kind of care I'm about to receive."

"Don't be ridiculous," Miriam said.

We walked out of the reception area and entered a series of wide, dark corridors that led to various departments. The radiology department consisted of an L-shaped hallway, flanked on both sides by larger rooms containing imaging machines. People sat on chairs in the hallway. Not knowing what to do, we sat down next to an elderly woman.

"Is there a waiting room?" I asked the woman.

"This is it," she replied. "Nice, eh?"

"I'm here for a PET scan. Do you know who I should I talk to?"

She pointed to a woman wearing a blue print nurse's smock.

I stood up and approached the nurse. "I'm Paul Stoller. I'm here for a ten-thirty PET scan."

She went into a room off the hallway and returned with a pile of papers. "Let's see," she said, thumbing through the documents. "Right." She looked at me. "Someone will be right with you."

I sat down next to Miriam, who had been reading a novel, her usual way of coping with hospital environments. Two volunteers pushed a gurney, carrying an ashen-faced young man to some imaging assignation. A frail-looking older woman fidgeted in her wheelchair. Other people waited patiently for loved ones who had disappeared into one of the image-making rooms. One robust man, perhaps sixty years old, was taken for a PET scan. His wife, who sat nearby, explained that he had been diagnosed with lung cancer.

"He was always full of life and energy. He worked hard and had just retired. . . . Now this."

A tall, lean young man finally called my name. "Would you come back with me?"

I entered one of the imaging rooms and sat down. He asked me some questions and pricked my finger to measure my blood sugar, which was normal. "We inject a radioactive glucose solution into you. When the cells process the sugar, we can see if the metabolic rate is normal or abnormal."

"I see," I said, gulping at the thought of a radioactive injection.

"We need to know if you've got normal blood sugar."

"Of course," I said, trying to appear brave.

He made some notations on a chart. "Follow me."

We walked down the hall to a small, dark room with two chairs and a bed.

"I need to get an IV going for the injection," he said. "Right or left?"

"Left," I said. If someone was going to inject me with a radioactive solution, I sure as hell wanted it to be on the left side!

Once the IV was properly inserted, he left. "I'll be right back with your injection."

Five minutes later he returned carrying a large black box.

"What's that?" I asked.

"It's a lead box. Your injection is inside."

"Why the lead box?" I asked.

"Well," he said, pausing, "it's radioactive."

"And you're injecting it into me!"

"Don't be alarmed," he added. "It's a very low dose and you'll eliminate it in twenty-four hours."

"That's reassuring," I said, eyeing the ominous-looking black box.

"You get limited exposure," he said gently. "I handle this stuff every day."

His words had the intended effect and I began to relax a bit.

"I'm going to give you the injection now. It may feel a little warm going in."

"Okay."

"You need to lie still for about forty-five minutes," he said when he'd finished. "We don't want unnecessary activity. That will increase your metabolism and can produce an inaccurate reading."

"I don't want that," I said.

"No, you don't," he said as he left the room, closing the door behind him.

It is not easy for anyone to sit completely still for forty-five minutes, especially if you are about to get scanned to see if cancer is still in your body. What to do with all that time? I tried to meditate. Breathing steadily and deeply, I visualized a midsummer beach on the Bay of Gibraltar in southern Spain that I had visited as a young man. A haze hovers over the bay; clouds enshroud much of the great rock. I see myself on the beach—thin, young, nearly penniless, and without a care in the world. The sun is strong and soothing. As my body beads with sweat, the calm tide gently caresses my feet with cool water—like being touched by the hand of God. With that image in mind, I dozed off only to be awakened by an attractive young woman with thick curly black hair. A gold cross was attached to a gold chain around her neck.

"Hi, I'm Diane. I'm going to do your PET scan. Do you want to get up and follow me?"

We walked down the hallway and turned right into a wider corridor. She looked at the restroom. "Do you have to go?"

I slipped into the men's room.

"Are you ready?" she asked as I emerged.

I nodded and suddenly we were outside. The PET scanner was housed in a large trailer. We climbed the steps and entered PET-scan land. To my right was a maze of computer equipment. To my left was the PET scanner, which looked a lot like the body-sucking CAT scanner. "Just like the CAT scan," I remarked.

"Yes," she said. "But with this you don't have to hold your breath or anything like that." I heard music from an oldies station. "Is that music okay?" she asked as she strapped me onto the gantry.

"It's the station I listen to."

"Good," she said. "This is going to take about forty minutes. You'll hear lots of noise from the machine. That means that it's taking pictures. Don't worry about the noise. Try to relax. There's nothing to it."

Nothing to it, I remarked silently, except that I have cancer and this machine is going to tell me if I'm in remission or not. The procedure was, in fact, much easier to bear than a CAT scan: no iodine contrast, no disembodied voice. I closed my eyes and again visualized a relaxing scene from my past. I'm walking amid enormous trees. As I near the top of a hill, I smell the scent of the ocean.

The technician tugged my arm. "We're finished," she said. "You got pretty relaxed in there, didn't ya?"

"I must have dozed off," I said, smiling.

"We've never had anyone fall asleep in the PET scanner!"

She accompanied me to the hallway waiting area. "You can wait and get your film in one hour or we can mail it to you."

"I'd prefer it if you'd mail them," I said, eager to leave the hospital.

She shook my hand and offered the usual "Good luck."

I went off to find Miriam. We left the sterile hospital environment and drove into the midday traffic of the "real world." Before going to work, we stopped for lunch at a small restaurant, which helped to restore our sense of normality.

After yet another interminable wait for the results of medical tests, I received the findings of the PET scan by fax from the staff at The Cancer Center. The radiologist who dictated the document—rarely, if ever, do they actually write up results—did so in a chillingly dispassionate way. My name was mentioned under the heading "Patient Name." After that I was referred to once as the "fifty-four-year-old male with a history of abdominal lymphoma." The document suggested a positive response to chemotherapy. The radiologist, however, couldn't say with certainty that I—"the subject"—had achieved complete remission. According to the radiologist: "Overall, the findings suggest an excellent tumor response to chemotherapy but require some form of follow-up to demonstrate long-term stability and PET scanning would be the most sensitive means for follow-up given the findings present on this examination and the presence of a residual soft tissue mass/scar on CAT examination."

Put in more accessible language, the whole-body PET scan was "unremarkable," meaning that the metabolic processes in my body had been normal—not malignant. The tumor, the radiologist wrote, was predominantly hypometabolic, which meant that it consisted of scar tissue, which signified, in turn, that there were no lymphoma cells lurking about. Even so, the radiologist found some "stippled uptake," a slight elevation of metabolic activity, at the tumor's center. The uptake could indicate surviving lymphoma cells. By the same token, the document suggested, the finding could have resulted from an inflammation caused by the interaction of toxic chemotherapy drugs with dead lymphoma cells at the tumor site. The radiologist also noted some subtle abnormalities in the stomach, which could have been caused by gastritis, an ulcer, or residual lymphoma cells. The stomach abnormalities might have also been an artifact—a false positive precipitated by the scanning process. If I—"the subject"—had clinical symptoms, the radiologist recommended an endoscopy—sticking a small camera-mounted tube down the esophagus to have a look-see at the stomach.

What can be more frustrating than to undergo a cutting-edge medical procedure only to learn that the results were inconclusive? That scenario might pique the interest of radiologists attempting to refine their interpretations of increasingly sensitive scanning technologies, but it leaves the poor cancer patient—me, in this instance—betwixt and between. There was unmistakable good news, but the good news might not be so good.[8] How ironic it seemed that increasing technological sophistication brought less rather than more diagnostic precision.

Two days later I brought the PET-scan report to Joel Rubin. After a short wait in one of The Cancer Center's small, dark, spare examination rooms, Joel came in carrying my ever expanding file.

We shook hands. "How have you been?"

"I've liked the break from the chemotherapy. I almost feel normal."

Joel smiled. "Normal is good."

"I read the report," I said. "These radiologists have a peculiar relationship with the English language."

"Yes they do," Joel admitted. "It's a pretty good report," he stated. "We have to decide what the next course should be. You're in partial remission, but there may be residual lymphoma cells in the center of the tumor. We could stop now."

"I don't want to take that chance," I said immediately. "If there's even the possibility of surviving lymphoma cells, I'd like to get rid of them."

"That's what I'd recommend." He jotted some notes. "Let's do three more cycles of chemotherapy and Rituxan and get another set of scans to see what gives. Is that okay?"

Having already decided that this was the best course of action, I nodded.

"I said at the beginning that it would take at least eight months of chemotherapy to bring you into remission," Joel added to remind me of the difficulty of eliminating slow-growing lymphoma from the body.

❀ ❀ ❀

Misery filled my life for the next nine weeks. I had downplayed the cumulative effects of chemotherapy drugs on the body. Throughout the first eight three-week cycles, I had ten bad days and eleven good days. I hadn't lost my hair and hadn't experienced bouts of nausea. Painful sores hadn't erupted in my mouth. Infections hadn't triggered fevers. My white and red blood cell levels remained pretty much within normal ranges. I hadn't lost or gained weight. Fatigue hadn't severely restricted my activities, which meant that I had been able to exercise moderately and travel abroad. I had continued to teach. I did suffer from numbness in the extremities—especially the fingers—and I tended to get painful cramps in both my feet and hands—an effect of vincristine, which brings on the cumulative neurological side effects that I had experienced.[9]

As I went through the last phase of chemotherapy, though, the going got tough—more bad than good days. I developed a periodic sore throat. A line of painful mouth sores developed on the blade of my tongue, making it difficult to swallow. My bones throbbed, and I developed such pulsing pain in my right knee, the site of a previous skiing injury, that I found it difficult to walk. Pain and restlessness made a good night's sleep a gift to be savored. Numbness became more and more noticeable in my feet and hands. Hand and foot cramps froze my joints in painful positions.

When I complained of these side effects to Joel Rubin, he reiterated the fact that chemotherapy's side effects were cumulative—especially the neurological ones. "You've got neuropathy," he said. "The more vincristine you get, the worse it gets."

"It's really bothering me," I complained.

"I know," he said. "If you were a concert violinist, I'd either reduce the dosage or take you off of it."

"I'm no violinist, and I can still use the computer."

"I know it's a nuisance, but the numbness you describe is fairly mild. I'd recommend that we continue with the vincristine."

Easy for him to say, I thought. Even so, I agreed with him. "Good. We'll do two more cycles and then get more CAT and PET scans."

I somehow managed to make it through the last six weeks of treatment. Dull aching pain became my ever present companion. Meditation soothed some of my stresses and frustrations. I made small offerings on the altar in my home and thought often about my life, especially time with Adamu Jenitongo. In my dreams, I'd see myself seated next to my teacher in the shade of his conical straw hut. He'd chew his kola and spit out the tobacco nested under his lip. He'd tell stories about ancestors who could fly great distances and subdue dangerous witches. He'd talk about how a person on sorcery's path must be patient. The world is patience, he'd say. *The world is patience.* Never before had I realized the importance of this adage. Adamu Jenitongo's presence brought me comfort. No matter the difficulty of my path, his words gave me the resolve to move forward with a degree of quiet confidence. My time with him had given me a glimpse into a world filled with pain and suffering. I had seen men and women of all ages face difficulties with strength and courage. The wisdom of Songhay sorcery provided these people a measure of solace and a degree of understanding. Although my own middle-class suburban American upbringing had paved the way for my professional life, it had not prepared me for the pain and suffering of cancer. Instead, the wisdom of Songhay sorcery helped me to deal with the devastation that cancer brings to life. It calmed me in stressful situations. It enabled me to be patient in circumstances that provoked impatience. It gave me strength and determination in times of physical and emotional distress. And, as odd as it may seem, it showed me how to incorporate cancer into my life so that I could use it to grow both physically and emotionally.

Finally, the last day of my treatment arrived. I took three bottles of champagne to the oncology nurses, who had been so kind to me. "You've looked after me wonderfully," I said. "This is one of my favorite champagnes. I hope you enjoy it." I paused a moment. "I give it to you with this African blessing: *Iri koy ma kati or se lafia.* May the High God bring you total peace."

The nurses, who were now used to my strange ways, hugged me and wished me good luck. I picked a chair and Jennifer hooked me up to what I hoped would be the last IV line I'd have to look at for a very long time.

"We have a happy hour this Friday," she said. "We'll drink the champagne then." She adjusted the flow of the medicines into my vein. "You know, Paul, you got things down pretty good. Every treatment session you brought the things that were important to you, your African cloth, a book, your music, and your funny stories. That's a good way to cope with treatment," she said. "It hasn't been easy, has it?"

"No, it hasn't," I said honestly.

"We'll miss you here."

"Thanks, but I'll be coming around for checkups from time

to time. I'll make sure to stop by and visit. You know, I hope to write a book about my experiences. You'll definitely be in it."

"I'll look forward to reading it," she said as she pushed a small dose of vincristine into the IV tube.

❀ ❀ ❀

Again I scheduled CAT and PET scans. The results would determine if I had, indeed, entered a state of complete remission. The results did, in fact, confirm a lymphoma-free state. The PET scan document contained the following finding: "Negative whole-body PET imaging.... No evidence of significant uptake of Fluorine-18 FDG is noted in the region of the mass in the root of the mesentery demonstrated on several CAT scans."

Several weeks later I had an appointment with Joel Rubin to discuss the scan results. He read the reports and smiled. "This is excellent: no visible or metabolic traces of lymphoma." He looked at me. "I think you're in complete remission," he said, holding out his hand. "Congratulations!"

"Thank you, Joel," I said as relief and joy coursed through me. I told myself that I would try to enjoy every moment of time given to me. "This calls for champagne."

Having lived in France, I had learned that champagne is not only offered to celebrate important occasions, but is also considered a healing tonic. My French friend Jean-Paul once told me that champagne was at one time served to patients recuperating from surgery.

"Good choice," he said as he added some notes to my file. "We can obviously stop treatment now," he said. "There are some choices you'll need to make. We'll need to monitor you. I'd like to see you in three months for a checkup. And you'll need to get a CAT scan every six months for the next few years."

"To see if the lymphoma returns."

"It does have that tendency," Joel admitted soberly.

"I know." Even this gloomy pronouncement did not bring my soaring spirits back to earth.

"You could also elect to get antibody treatment in six months. We don't have very much clinical evidence, but Rituxan could knock out any stray lymphoma that the scans didn't pick up. That could extend remission," he said. "You could get a series of treatments, one a week for six weeks."

"I think I'd like to do that," I said.

"Minimal side effects with a very positive potential," Joel stated. "I'd do it."

We spoke then about the uncertainties of remission, the likelihood of the cancer returning. After a short while Joel said, "This is a good day. Let's keep the focus positive. You're in remission. Go get your champagne and celebrate."

CHAPTER FOUR

Remissioning Life

On the day that I entered remission I bought several bottles of Cordon Rouge. I invited Miriam and several other friends to my apartment to celebrate. Once we had all assembled, I proposed a toast: "To years of health and happiness." The champagne tasted cool, sharp, and delicious. As I filled the flutes for the second time, I wondered about the meaning of the toast I had just proposed: how many years of health, exactly? How long could I expect to remain in remission? Joel Rubin had not been able to answer that question when I posed it to him earlier that day at The Cancer Center.

"You could be in remission for two years, five years. In some cases, people remain in remission for ten years. In other cases, the lymphoma comes back after six months, which would be terrible."

"I'm really in uncharted territory then," I stated.

"I'm afraid so. You'll need to get CAT scans to monitor your condition. Let's hope that they show stability. Let's hope they show that the disease hasn't progressed."

"Remission is a difficult path to follow," I said.

Joel nodded.

The term *remission* comes from the verb *to remit*, which can refer to, among other things, states of relief, abatement, hiatus, interruption, respite, stoppage, and subsidence. Except for stoppage, none of the states connoted by *remission* signifies a condition of permanence. Such words as *relief, abatement, interruption, respite,* and *subsidence* suggest an eventual return to a preexisting state. *Hiatus* refers to a temporary place between what was and what will be. Even *stoppage* betrays an indirect impermanence. In the end, remission means spending years "being on hold," "waiting for the other shoe to drop," or "sitting on your hands." It is not an easy place to be.[1]

Entering the state of remission prompted me to think about Claude Levi-Strauss's classic work, *Tristes Tropiques*, a memoir that tells the story of Levi-Strauss's first field mission to Brazil in the 1930s. It is a book filled with sensuous descriptions of the tropics as well as brilliant observations about the human condition. One chapter, called "The Doldrums," evocatively captures the personal significance of going to an exotic land to conduct an anthropological field study. On a steamer en route to Brazil, Levi-Strauss writes about what it is like to sail through a zone in the Atlantic—"the doldrums"—where the northerly trade winds end and the southerly trade winds have yet to begin. In a memorable passage, this distinguished anthropologist writes about how storms form at the edge of the doldrums. Stationed at the deck rail of the ship, he describes the slow buildup of black storm clouds, which eventually bear down on the steamer only to suddenly stop as if they had hit an invisible wall. Then the clouds curiously "turn around" and move back toward the north. Observing this bizarre weather pattern compelled Levi-Strauss to think what it would have been like to negotiate the doldrums in an eighteenth-century sailing vessel. In that time the doldrums were a point of no return. Once in this zone, wind patterns made a quick return to the familiar and comforting life of the Old World exceedingly difficult. Caught in the dead calm of the doldrums, travelers had to slowly proceed south and west.

Eventually, ships caught a southwesterly trade wind that propelled them toward unknown worlds in which alien peoples spoke exotic languages. Although most travelers would eventually return home, Levi-Strauss suggests, experiences in the New World would forever change their perception of the Old World.

When cancer patients enter the zone of remission, it is not unlike negotiating the doldrums. You are in a space between the comfortable assumptions of your old life and the uncomfortable uncertainties of your new life. You have long left the village of the healthy in which sickness is a temporary respite from good health. Once you enter the village of the sick, as I have suggested, you can never fully return to the village of the healthy.

During chemotherapy, you reside deep within the village of the sick. The routine of treatments and side effects consumes your conscious thoughts and soaks up your time. When you reach remission, however, you are not unlike Claude Levi-Strauss's eighteenth-century traveler on a voyage to the New World. Having regained your equilibrium, you have the energy to walk to the gate of your new village. From your vantage you see the open gate to the village of the healthy. In your state of "respite," you can leave the domain of sickness and walk the short distance to the space of health. People there know you and greet you. Even so, you realize that you have changed. People talk to you and wish you well, but you quickly understand that your time in the village of the sick has set you apart. You desperately want to live again in the village of the healthy, but sadly understand that your place is elsewhere. In the village of the healthy, you are surrounded by friends and family, but often feel alone. In the village of the sick, a way station on your journey, you are surrounded by strangers, but are silently bonded to them. They know what you know.

Seen in this light, remission is an example of what anthropologists have called "liminality." The late Victor Turner, one of the most influential anthropologists of the twentieth century, wrote extensively about the liminal state. "Liminal entities," he wrote in his book *The Ritual Process,* "are neither here nor there; they are betwixt and between the positions assigned and arrayed by custom, convention, and ceremonial" (p. 95). People in liminal states tend to be humble. They usually do what they are told to do—often without complaint. They accept regimens of pain. They are reduced to a common denominator so that they might be reconstructed. These processes create an intense camaraderie, which washes away previously recognized differences in age, social status, and ethnicity. Turner called this camaraderie "communitas."

Liminality is a common phenomenon in human experience. It is a central feature of what anthropologists call "rites of passage." A rite of passage is a ceremony that marks a transitional event in the life cycle: birth, initiation, marriage, death. Before an initiation rite, for example, young boys and girls are considered children. During initiation, they receive specialized training about hunting, farming, sexuality, and religion. During this period of liminal training, groups of initiates, who are now considered neither children nor adults, are often isolated in sacred spaces reserved for the learning of important and powerful secrets. At the end of training, ceremonies are performed that mark the transition from childhood to adulthood. In some societies, this transition is marked by circumcision or ritual scarification. In a few societies neophytes are literally buried. They leave their childhood in mock graves and arise from them as full-fledged adults.

In the Jewish tradition the bar or bat mitzvah is a rite of passage that comprises all of these ritual properties. Before the bar or bat mitzvah ceremony, boys and girls are considered children. They cannot fully participate in Jewish religious activities. Several years before the transitional ceremony, religious specialists not only verse them in the history and principles of the Jewish tradition, but also teach them to read and write Hebrew. They go to Hebrew school, an experience that they share with other neophytes in the spirit of communitas. In time, they are ready to demonstrate their competence before a congregation. During the ceremony, they recite prayers in Hebrew and give a speech about what it means to come of age in the Jewish tradition. At the end of the ceremony, either a Friday night or Saturday morning Sabbath service, the rabbi acknowledges the neophyte's new status as an adult member of the religious community.

In many ways cancer patients are very much liminal figures in society. Like neophytes, cancer patients are often socially set apart by stereotypical images: a pallor, a hairless head, a shuffling walk, a skeletal body. These are images of impending death. Given our intense fear of death in American society, people who trigger these images do not fit into the routine of prescribed social patterns. Like many neophytes, cancer patients also submit to a regimen of pain—chemotherapy, which they usually receive in infusion rooms. These spaces are often arranged to encourage informal talk and camaraderie. Communitas may or may not develop in the infusion room, but cancer patients who are in or have completed treatment—"survivors"—are encouraged to participate in support groups.[2] Bonded by the cancer experience, strangers feel comfortable enough to express their fears—of pain and death—to one another in ways that would make an "outsider" uncomfortable. From a liminal vantage, these encounters are part of "survival" training, a way of making treatment and remission easier to bear.

There is, however, a twist to the cancer patient's liminality. For most neophytes liminality is a transitional state. Most people are in liminal states for only short periods of time, after which they are reintegrated into society. After spending months in a West African sacred forest where they learn the secrets of the hunt, teenaged boys look forward to returning to their villages as young men. When they return home they are no longer liminal figures—no longer betwixt and between. What can the liminal cancer patient look forward to? During treatment, you look forward to the end of chemotherapy and its debilitating side effects. At that point, you are in remission, which continues rather than ends your liminality. The twist, then, is that the liminality of the cancer patient may subside, but it rarely ends. Even though you are feeling fine, there is, for all intents and purposes, no full-fledged return to the village of the healthy.

Cancer patients, of course, are not the only people who live in a continuous state of liminality. Consider the lives of immigrants. They leave their ancestral homes and settle in new lands in which the language is foreign and the customs are exotic. Even if immigrants have a long history in their adopted lands, they may not truly feel at home. Even if they return to the land of their birth, their experience overseas will have changed them. They will see home through different eyes; concomitantly, the people at home will also see them differently. These dynamics, which may make the immigrant feel out of sorts, sets a course of continuous liminality.

Sorcerers are the masters of liminality. Among the Songhay, sorcerers live in shadow lands where life is more than what it seems, where one must be prepared to walk with great care and purpose. They wander in the space where the social and spirit worlds intersect. As they move forward, they must continuously think about the liminal space they inhabit. One careless move can have devastating consequences. They are, to paraphrase Victor Turner, neither here nor there. Given the uncertainties of the sorcerer's life and the mysteries of his or her power, people try their best to avoid these "spiritual guardians." Upon seeing the approach of a sorcerer, Songhay might walk the other way. Most Songhay villagers choose to live far away from the sorcerer's family—lest they be burned by the sorcerer's unbridled power. Adamu Jenitongo lived at the edge of Tillaberi, a compound situated between the violent bush and the peaceful village. Adamu Jenitongo thrived in liminal space.

How did he do it? Like remission, continuous liminality is hard to bear. You are always marked as an outsider. Many people go out of their way to avoid you. When you do interact with others, they often avoid bringing up certain subjects. Beyond these limitations, continuous liminality offers no conclusion, only more treacherous terrain to negotiate. Like most Songhay sorcerers, Adamu Jenitongo confronted his continuous liminality with pragmatic wisdom, especially when he lived for twenty years in French prison camps in the Sahara Desert—spaces of continuous liminality par excellence.

❊ ❊ ❊

When he was in his mid-forties, Adamu Jenitongo was arrested by the French authorities, accused of killing a man who had become his wife's lover. Supposedly, Adamu Jenitongo confronted the man in the bush and cut his head off. The French administration convicted him. Classified as a dangerous criminal, the colonial court sentenced Adamu Jenitongo to life in prison. He spent several years in the Tillaberi prison in Niger, where he worked on road gangs and toiled in the gardens of the commandant of the Department of Tillaberi. At the outbreak of World War II, the French transferred their most dangerous criminals to a bleak outpost in the southern Sahara, where prisoners were forced to work under dire conditions. Many prisoners died at this infamous prison camp, Bidon 5. On several occasions, Adamu Jenitongo thought that he, too, would die alone in the desert. Accepting his limitations, he began to use sorcerous knowledge to improve his situation. Whenever his French captors complained of losing something, Adamu Jenitongo volunteered his services: "I'll find it for you."

Soon the French officers came to him with a variety of requests. Adamu Jenitongo performed these services with economy and good humor. He found money that they had lost. He

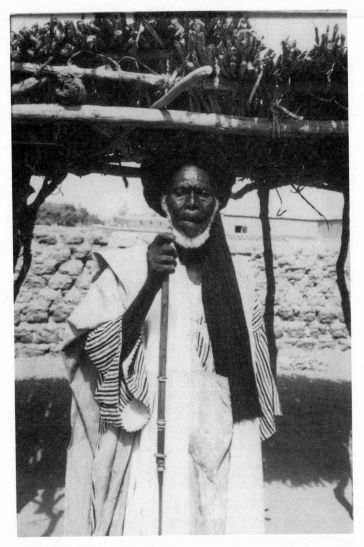

Adamu Jenitongo in his Tillaberi, Niger, compound (1987). Photo: Paul Stoller

gave them herbs to make them feel better. The French officers moved him to better quarters and soon made him the chef of the officer's mess, which meant that Adamu Jenitongo's diet improved considerably. At the end of the war, Adamu Jenitongo was transferred to the prison at Chidal. Situated along one of two major trans-Saharan routes, Chidal was bigger, even luxurious, in comparison with Bidon 5. Adamu Jenitongo quickly installed himself in the officer's kitchen.

"I've never seen so much meat, potatoes, and cabbage," he told me years later. "The officers ate well. So did I!"

He continued to perform minor sorcerous services for the French officers as well as his fellow prisoners. He found lost objects. He cured African inmates of spirit sicknesses. He administered herbal medicines to local French families. In time the French entrusted him with their children. Having accepted his limitations, Adamu Jenitongo used what he knew to make the prisoner's life as sweet as it could be. He remained at Chidal for another fifteen years. When France granted the Republic of Niger its independence in 1960, the officers at Chidal freed Adamu Jenitongo. By then in his late seventies, he sent a telegram to his sister, Kedibo, asking her to meet him at the Tillaberi bus depot.

During his years in prison, Adamu Jenitongo's rich diet of meat and potatoes had made him so fat that his sister did not recognize him.

"How did you get so big?" she asked when she saw her brother for the first time in more than twenty years.

"I ate meat and potatoes every day," he replied.

"Adamu," his brother-in-law said, "we thought you were dead. And now you're here—fat and prosperous."

"I thank God," replied Adamu Jenitongo.

"You need to find a wife," he said. "My sister is a good young woman. Why not marry her?"

Adamu married his brother-in-law's sister and even, as was customary, took a second wife from his home region of Zarmagunda. By 1964, he had established himself on his dunetop compound. People came to recognize him as a great sorcerer and spirit-possession priest.[3] He spent the rest of his life happily helping those who came to him.

❁ ❁ ❁

Adamu Jenitongo's narrative underscores how Songhay sorcerers deal with a state of continuous liminality. Realizing that death had become his close neighbor at Bidon 5, Adamu Jenitongo assessed his "hopeless" situation and took small, pragmatic steps to improve his situation. Although he had the capacity to punish or even kill some of his captors, he realized that such action would hinder rather than help him—and, for that matter, his fellow prisoners. And so he performed small feats that won the grudging admiration of the French prison officials. Although he remained a prisoner in a prison camp—the epitome of a liminal figure—he thrived in a hostile environment. He found comfort in uncomfortable circumstances.

When you are diagnosed with cancer and undergo a regimen of chemotherapy, you confront, like Adamu Jenitongo, a set of adverse circumstances. You don't have to be a Songhay sorcerer to meet these circumstances head-on. I have discussed some of the things that helped me to adjust to the uncertainty of diagnosis and the pain of treatment—playing my favorite music, wearing "lucky" clothes, bringing objects that made the infusion room seem more like home.

Remission, though, is a trickier enterprise than is treatment. At the end of treatment, the side effects of chemotherapy drugs slowly fade away. The aches and pains dissipate. The mouth sores disappear. Your throat clears. The fevers fade away. Your appetite returns. Energy surges through your body. Even though you feel "normal," you still think about cancer every day—if only for a little while. Like Adamu Jenitongo at Bidon 5, you understand that cancer is a traveler who may appear on your doorstep at any moment. How do you confront a life that cancer has complicated and perhaps shortened? Once in remission, some cancer patients become bitter and resentful.[4] Others try to conquer their adversary. Like Fran Dresher, the actress, they say "cancer shmancer," the phrase that is the title of Dresher's 2002 book on "surviving" breast cancer. In this approach, which is much admired in American culture, cancer patients pummel their enemy into submission, forcing it into the background of their consciousness. This willfulness may well enable some people to lead full lives during remission—at least until remission ends.

Taking into consideration individual differences in how people react to sickness, Songhay culture promotes a much less individualistic approach to illness and death. Finding themselves in the shadows cast by the natural forces of life and death, the Songhay are taught to think that they are relatively insignificant beings—trickles, as I have stated, in the stream of history. Swept up in the strong current of life, many Songhay think that life is like a loan that can never fully be repaid. On the given due date, you must make a payment, but you can never pay off the principle. You hope that your payments make a lasting contribution to your family, friends, and community. This type of cultural orientation breeds considerable respect for the forces of the universe, including the ongoing presence of illness in the body. If a Songhay develops a serious illness like cancer, he or she is likely to build respect for it. Respect for cancer—or any illness—does not mean that you meekly submit to the ravages of disease. Following the ideas of sages like Adamu Jenitongo, illness is accepted as an ongoing part of life. When illness appears, it presents one with limitations, but if it is possible to accept the limitations and work within their parameters, one can, like Adamu Jenitongo, create a degree of comfort in uncomfortable circumstances. Adamu Jenitongo incorporated prison into his being. He thrived during a more than twenty-year period of incarceration. The same logic can be extended to cancer. By incorporating cancer into your being, you can, like the cyclist Lance Armstrong, use it to creatively build strength and endurance. Had Armstrong not gone through cancer diagnosis and treatment, would he have become a seemingly invincible cycling champion?

Adamu Jenitongo long ago accepted the limitations that

continuous liminality brings. In so doing, he purged himself of resentment. When the French freed him after more than twenty years in prison, he harbored no resentment toward his captors. Indeed, he left Chidal on good terms and returned to Niger ready to resume his life as a healer and spiritual guardian. In his second life, Adamu Jenitongo, like Lance Armstrong, performed remarkable feats. His case is not an isolated one. Nelson Mandela lived for more than twenty-five years in a South African prison. Despite the rigors of his confinement, prison life, which Mandela incorporated into his being, created in him an unimpeachable dignity. As a free man, he bore no hatred toward white South Africans. In the absence of resentment, he united a nation torn by years of civil strife and social atrocity.

Remission can also be like a prison from which the cancer patient cannot escape. Confronting remission's impermanence is not easy. There are junctures during remission that remind you what a delicate state it can be. Once in remission, waiting for the results of regularly scheduled CAT scans can become exceedingly stressful and can plunge you into depression. If the results come back normal, remission continues. If the scans indicate the return of malignant cells, you may need an additional, more powerfully toxic treatment. You may even need palliative care to ease the journey toward your ultimate demise, which is, of course, a destination we all share.

Remission has been difficult for me. Although I have suggested many ideas that can ease the burden of remission, I do not for a minute pretend to have foolproof solutions to the quandaries it presents. My experiences in the world of Songhay sorcery have helped me to cope with the diagnosis of and treatment for lymphoma. What's more, Adamu Jenitongo's soft voice comes to me regularly in dreams. He reminds me to accept my limitations and remove resentment from my mind. He tells me to be patient in a world of impatience. He encourages me to be humble and refine my knowledge so that others might learn from it. His strong presence in my life, however, has not completely extinguished my fears. If I have a twinge in my abdomen, I fear that lymphoma cells are again on the rampage. If an ingrown hair causes a bump to develop in my armpit, I think it may be a swollen lymph node—another sign of lymphoma. If the flu makes me sweat at night, I worry that this too is a sign that cancer has returned. When I get a CAT scan every six months I wonder if my time is up.

The wisdom of Songhay sorcerers is not a panacea for cancer patients. But the wisdom of men and women who face more difficult lives than we do is instructive. Remission is exceedingly stressful, but its stressful junctures are few and far between. Like Adamu Jenitongo, it helps to accept remission's limitations and seize the moment. In so doing, you can acknowledge that our time on earth is borrowed and that a central mission in life is to contribute knowledge—whatever that may be or entail—to our families, friends, colleagues, and communities. In so doing, is it not possible to squeeze some sweet pleasure from life?

CHAPTER FIVE

Bearing Witness on the Wings of the Wind

Cancer is a devastating collection of more than one hundred different diseases. These diseases have one thing in common. They consist of malignant cells that grow inexorably into tumors that block blood flow, restrict the movement of essential fluids, precipitate internal organ failure, or, in the case of some blood cancers, cells that destroy the immune system. The growth of these cells causes much pain and suffering. They usually bring on death.

More often than not, cancers grow slowly and silently. Except for skin cancers, they grow invisibly in the body—in the bowels, ovaries, prostate, liver, kidneys, lungs, in breast tissue, the brain, and the blood—to name the most prominent sites—until symptoms suggest the presence of malignancy. Such devastating invisibility promotes fear—even of the word *cancer*. For most of us, going back to Susan Sontag's memorable work, cancer is an unspeakable evil. It is like an alien that slowly and relentlessly takes over the body. When we find this mortal enemy hiding in our viscera, we submit to toxic treatments that aim to purge the body of its alien foe. Despite the complex perseverance of cancer, treatments are becoming more and more effective. There is increasing talk of "surviving" cancer. There is even a realistic expectation of eventually "winning the war" against this pernicious collection of diseases. Attempting to "win the war" against illness, as I have suggested, is a quintessentially American approach to disease.

In the preceding pages, I have attempted to present an alternative view of cancer. Shaped by non-Western conceptions of illness and disease, it is an orientation that incorporates rather than destroys illness-in-the-body. Following the insights of David Napier in his book *The Age of Immunology,* the incorporation of illness does not mean that a person submits to her or his disease and morosely awaits death. It does mean that you use the experience of disease positively—to grow and change. For most Americans, including myself, this lesson is a hard one to accept. Before cancer appeared in my body, I considered disease a nuisance that had to treated and eradicated. I subscribed fully to the view that illness is an enemy that had to be quickly annihilated. I maintained this orientation to illness even though I had lived many years among a West African people who held very different beliefs about illness and health. I sustained a militaristic view of illness despite long training in Songhay sorcery, which seeks to master illness through incorporation rather than defeat.

When cancer presented itself in my body, its terrifying presence forced me to think deeply about the relation of health and illness; it compelled me to ponder seriously my own death. Despite my stubborn resistance, having cancer prompted me to reconsider the course of my life. It brought me back to Songhay sorcery and, to again borrow from T. S. Eliot, "to know the place for the first time." I realized that I had had only a superficial grasp of the deeper meanings of Songhay sorcerous practices. Cancer focused my attention away from the superficial rivalries that had marked my early travels on sorcery's path and redirected my gaze to its pragmatic wisdom. Having discovered these deeper realities, I attempted to use the pragmatic wisdom of Songhay sorcery to cope with the physical and emotional pain of the diagnosis and treatment of cancer. More recently I have tried to extend Songhay ideas to cope with remission.

My story, of course, is by no means unique, for experience is a great teacher. We cannot understand certain events or emotions until we are ready to. Consider the experience of the anthropologist Renato Resaldo, who studied the Ilongot headhunters of the Philippines. In books and essays, he probed their culture and analyzed their history. He attempted to use various social theories to explain how Ilongot grief prompted rage that, in turn, compelled headhunting. In a celebrated essay, "Grief and the Headhunter's Rage," he tells the story of how his wife, Michelle Zimbalist Rosaldo, who like her husband was a highly respected anthropologist, fell to her death during a field expedition in the Philippines. Responding to her tragic death, Rosaldo felt for the first time the emotional depth of Ilongot grief and the headhunter's rage. Through his unexpected confrontation with sudden death, Rosaldo broadened his cultural understanding and deepened his humanity. In the same vein, if lymphoma cells had not colonized part of my abdomen, I seriously doubt that I would have revisited sorcery's path and grasped for the first time a few of its deeper meanings.

Cancer has not only had a profound impact on my understanding of sorcery, but also on my professional life as a social scientist. When I attended graduate school in the 1970s, social science generated a great deal of excitement in the academy. At that time mainstream social scientists, including anthropologists, believed that they could discover the universal principles that governed social behavior. Many anthropologists thought that if they carefully examined the structures of societies, they would uncover "deep" rules that would explain the inner workings of social life. Other scholars, following the lead of the aforementioned Claude Levi-Strauss, believed that the comparative study of art, myth, and kinship would reveal universal principles of cognition. These, in turn, would unlock the mystery of how people think. Focusing on ritual life, a school of anthropologists concentrated their efforts on how people use symbols to construct their cultures. Considering the complexities of everyday routine interaction, yet another group of anthropologists and sociologists analyzed conversational practices among other taken-for-granted actions to isolate "rules" that governed behavior. No matter the approach that scholars took to understanding the complexities of social life, they believed that they could use a variety of theories to get to the bottom of things. Through systematic analysis, scholars, it was believed, could peel away the superficialities of social reality and reveal explanatory truth. Like their colleagues in the natural sciences, anthropologists followed what John Dewey called "the quest for certainty," the attempt to convert social chaos to cultural order.

The drive toward universality, however, brought on discontent. Could you extract order from chaos? Would it not be more realistic to describe "thickly," to borrow from the anthropologist Clifford Geertz, the ever complex multilayered textures of social life? To paraphrase a famous Geertzian quip, the closer you get to the bottom of things, the more confusing those things become. Disenchanted with the dehumanized search for human universals, Geertz advocated what he called the "thick description" of social life in which culture is considered as a text. The anthropological challenge in Geertz's universe was to develop the capacity—over time—to "read" and sensitively interpret the textual properties of social and cultural life. In time, anthropologists could write books that did not reduce society or culture to a series of rules, but represented more fully the inexplicable complexity of social and cultural life.

This mosaic of ideas presented me with an embarrassment of riches. Which orientation to social and cultural life would suit my sensibilities? Because I wanted to return to West Africa, where I had been a Peace Corps volunteer, I wondered which orientation would provide the best tool for understanding West African societies. In preparation for my first field mission to Niger in 1976, I read the works of the French anthropologist and filmmaker Jean Rouch, who documented in books and films the social and cultural life of the Songhay people of Niger—the very people I proposed to study. Rouch's work impressed me in two ways. First, Rouch, like Geertz, foregrounded "thick" description and backgrounded explanatory theories. Second, he produced evocative and challenging films that underscored the dignity and wisdom of the Songhay. In his books and films Rouch demonstrated that Songhay people possessed knowledge not yet known to us. This theme represented a healthy dose of clear-sighted academic modesty.

After conducting a year of field research among the Songhay I returned to the United States to defend my dissertation. Although I wanted to write evocatively about the Songhay, the members of my doctoral committee gently advised me to link my thick descriptions to social theory in the hope that my work might make a contribution to the discipline. I made the suggested revisions and received my doctorate.

I continued to travel to Niger almost every year to immerse myself in the study of Songhay sorcery and spirit possession. As I began to write about my experiences in Niger, I sought some kind of intellectual justification for writing texts that were more evocative than most anthropological works. I wanted people to sense the texture of social life among the Songhay, but felt I needed to defend this textual choice. Accordingly I read the works of French philosophers like Maurice Merleau-Ponty, Jacques Derrida, Jean-François Lyotard, and Roland Barthes, as well as the equally impressive works of their American interpreters. These thinkers, especially Derrida, critiqued the idea of universal objective truth. They also suggested that the search for ultimate truth had, in part, triggered the emergence of totalitarian regimes in the twentieth century. This body of thought profoundly influenced my writing, in which I attempted to link narrative and theory. Writing in this way reinforced my commitment to social theories that linked global forces to local realities. Although I believed that it is the social scientist's mission to at least try to figure out "how things work" in social worlds, I did not believe that this should be achieved by giving short shrift to the people who inhabit these worlds.

When I confronted the reality of cancer, though, my perception of the anthropological odyssey shifted. Why had I devoted so much time and effort to writing about "how things work?" I had tried very hard to come to terms with the mysteries of spirit possession and sorcery. I had grappled with issues of how to write about social life. Despite my long-standing efforts, the results of my research, like the quandaries of social life, had been inconclusive. Considering these inconclusive results, why did I persist? Like most writers, I wanted my ideas discussed and debated. Like most anthropologists, I wanted disciplinary recognition. Like most scholars, I wanted to make contributions to knowledge.

Faced with a disease that can be "managed" but not "cured," I began to wonder about my obligations as an anthropologist. Should I continue to try to refine social theory? Should I continue to write "thickly" described stories? Cancer has shifted my sense of priorities. I now believe that the anthropologist's fundamental obligation is to use her or his repertoire of skills to bear witness. In so doing we are compelled to tell stories about kinship as well as cancer that shed light on social realities. As witnesses to social life, we are obliged to make our stories accessible so that a wide range of readers might discuss and debate what we have written. This shift may harmonize the bush at a cancer center, infuse an infusion room with a touch or warmth, or make the emotional instabilities of remission a bit easier to bear. In the end this turn may take us to that elusive and oft forgotten end of scholarship: wisdom, the knowledge that enables us to live well in the world.

❀ ❀ ❀

At the beginning of this book I suggested that cancer opened a pathway to my personal growth and development. I said that cancer had toughened my body and strengthened my resolve. Cancer, I stated, had also made me more realistic about the symbiotic relationship between illness and health. Confronting cancer, I wrote, helped to integrate my spiritual beliefs.

The idea that cancer or other life-threatening illnesses can be an unexpected opportunity for personal growth and development is not new. Any number of authors have discussed how serious illness inspired them to fruitfully change directions and deepen their sensibilities.[1] As these testaments suggest, it sometimes takes a deep shock to see what stands directly in front of us. What is less clear, however, is how illness shapes this new awareness. How does illness, which is our continuous companion, enable us to see things as clearly as the seasoned Songhay sorcerer?

There is obviously no absolute answer to this question, for each person's experience in the world is unique. In my case cancer seems to have had an unexpected integrative effect. It has enabled me to understand that my life has consisted of three previously unintegrated strands: childhood immersion into the culture of Judaism; assimilation into the culture of anthropology and social science; and initiation into the culture of Songhay sorcery.

As a child my parents immersed me in the culture of Judaism. I attended Hebrew school and was bar mitzvahed at the age of thirteen. At that point I ended my formal Jewish education. From then on I thought more about the institutions of Judaism than about its philosophic values, social responsibilities, and penchant for remembrance. As a young man, my graduate education assimilated me to the culture of anthropology. I learned how to write research proposals, conduct ethnographic research, and "write up" the results. I have been a professional anthropologist for more than twenty-five years, and yet during this span of years, I have spent little time wondering about how the culture of Judaism might have influenced my professional development. When I was a young anthropologist, Adamu Jenitongo initiated me into the culture of Songhay sorcery. I learned to mix potions, read divinatory shells, and recite incantations. Despite this rich set of experiences, I did not build bridges that seriously connected my apprenticeship in Songhay sorcery to either the culture of anthropology or the culture of Judaism. After the publication of *In Sorcery's Shadow* in 1987, I wrote little about sorcery "from the inside" for fear of professional ridicule. And rarely, if ever, did I think about how sorcery and Judaism might be connected in my life.

Confronting cancer forced me to integrate these disparate strands of my life. Having been diagnosed with and treated for lymphoma forced me to reflect deeply about the meaning of my life. This process compelled me to reconsider my life from an integrative vantage. Significant mentors like Adamu Jenitongo and Jean Rouch have inspired much of my work as an anthropologist. My works about them have been labors of remembrance. I attempted to write about these great figures so that their wisdom might be more deeply and widely appreciated. The will to remember and contribute to the world, I now realize, stems, in part, from my immersion in Jewish culture. My journey as an anthropologist, I have come to realize, gave me a way to appreciate both the ethical underpinnings of my upbringing as well as the philosophical foundation of sorcery. Even so, my Jewish upbringing and anthropological odyssey left a spiritual thirst in my life. Apprenticeship in Songhay sorcery quenched that thirst. By empowering me to integrate the disparate strands of my life, cancer showed me a way to growth and development that would have been impossible had my life proceeded as it had in the past.

It is unthinkable to be grateful for a diagnosis of cancer. No one desires the pain and suffering that come with a serious illness. But once you've got it, so to speak, why not incorporate it, as the Songhay would say, to bring to your being a deeper understanding of life's forces and meanings? Cancer can be used, and my example is one of many thousands, to grow and change. It can show you how to fly on the wings of the wind.[2]

Notes

1. The notion of the villages of the healthy and the sick are anthropological adaptations of Susan Sontag's more religious invocations of the "Kingdom of the Healthy and Kingdom of the Sick" in her book *Illness as Metaphor* (1978). The idea of a village of the sick is also similar to Arthur W. Frank's notion of the remission society, which he introduces in his second book, *The Wounded Storyteller: Body, Illness, and Ethics* (1995). Members of the remission society are people who "are effectively, but could never be considered cured. . . . Members of the remission society include those who have had almost any cancer, those living in cardiac recovery programs, diabetics, those whose allergies and environmental sensitivities require dietary and other self-monitoring, those with prostheses and mechanical body regulators, the chronically ill, the disabled, those 'recovering' from abuses and addictions, and for those people, the families that share the worries and daily triumph of staying well" (p. 8).

2. See Stoller (1989b, 1997, 1998).

3. Books on sorcery have a long history and many of them have been highly successful. Millions of readers have savored Carlos Castaneda's books on Don Juan Matus. Lynn Andrews's books on her studies with Native American healers have also sold well and widely. There is an equal fascination with North American witchcraft and paganism. Although *Stranger in the Village of the Sick* takes note of the kind of dramatic and mind-bending feats that have been described by Castaneda, and by myself in *In Sorcery's*

Shadow, its focus is on the practical wisdom of (Songhay) sorcery. In this way it extends the fascinating details—stories of sorcerers and their practices—of a sorcerous world and applies them practically and concretely to the world of cancer.

4. Cancer patients are no strangers to the memoir. They have published numerous personal accounts of how they coped with the quandaries of these diseases. The worst of these employ a "this is what happened to me" narrative style. Such "survivor" narratives have in recent times found a place on the Internet. They are featured on such Web sites as Oncolink, the Leukemia and Lymphoma Society, and on various discussion lists geared to particular kinds of cancer. In these electronic spaces, a cancer survivor can exchange her or his story with other patients—a way of encouraging others and extending hope.

The best cancer memoirs, in my view, are those in which authors have used their illness experience as a framework for broader discussion. Susan Sontag's award-winning *Illness as Metaphor* immediately comes to mind. In that book, a rather academic and historically focused work, Sontag employs "cancer" as the framework for a historical and literary discussion of the social categorization of illness. Stuart Alsop's memorable *Stay of Execution* is a riveting account of his confrontation with a particularly virulent form of leukemia. In addition to providing a memorable account of how it feels to be afflicted with leukemia, he uses his experience to reflect on such broadly based issues as courage, sacrifice, patriotism, World War II, and the demise of the East Coast WASP establishment. Arthur Frank's *At the Will of the Body* is a short memoir of the author's experience of illness (both heart disease and cancer) and renewal. Frank uses his experience in the "village of the sick" to suggest ways that patients can make sense of illness. He also uses his memoir to argue for more aggressive patient advocacy.

Stranger in the Village of the Sick differs significantly from these fine books. Unlike *Illness as Metaphor,* it is not an intellectual exercise about the sociological costs of our metaphoric categorization of illness. Unlike *Stay of Execution,* it is not an extended reflection upon the richness of life experience. Like *At the Will of the Body,* it does use the personal experience of cancer as a way to make sense of illness. *Stranger in the Village of the Sick,* however, juxtaposes African sorcery and cancer in order to suggest practical paths that, if followed, might improve the quality of a person's life.

5. The classic work on African sorcery remains E. E. Evans-Pritchard's *Witchcraft, Oracles and Magic among the Azande* (1937), a book more about

the logic of sorcerous beliefs than about the "reality" of sorcerous practices. This text generated a great deal of debate—ongoing—about the rationality of "apparently irrational beliefs" (see Sperber 1985). These debates, though, steer clear of the putative ontology of sorcery, or the effectiveness of sorcerous acts. In this way, the scholarly debates maintain a healthy—and skeptical—distance from more popular works that celebrate the "supernatural" aspects of sorcery. See also Wilson (1970). For an overview of the rationality debates, see Stoller (1998).

6. There is a vast literature, especially in sociolinguistics, on the power dynamics of doctor-patient communication. Among the best studies is Nancy Ainsworth-Vaughn's *Claiming Power in Doctor-Patient Talk* (1998), which analyzes how a position of power is achieved in such exchanges. In previous studies, Ainsworth-Vaughn claims, the asymmetry of medical discourse focused on the empowering conversational tactics of doctors. In Ainsworth-Vaughn's study, the focus is on how patients can seize power. "Doctors can do enormous good or enormous harm by what they say, and there are many books (virtually all the other books regarding provider-patient talk) that focus on what should and should not be said by providers to help bring about healing. But I think that medical education in the United States often implies that only providers are healers. Doctors and nurses who accept this idea take on an unnecessary burden. . . . Patients, too, have enormous contributions to make to their own well-being" (p. 189). See also Shuy (1993), Fisher (1986), and Fisher and Todd (1993).

7. Positron emission tomography (PET) scanning is a new imaging technology that "compares the differences in metabolic activity in abnormal tissue, such as cancerous tumors, to that of normal tissues, to produce an image of the location and possible spread of the tumor in the body. Other imaging modalities such as CAT, MRI, Ultrasound and x-ray rely on differences in structure and anatomy to separate normal and abnormal tissues. The PET scanner's unique ability to image differences in metabolic activity has proven to be more sensitive and specific, and therefore more accurate, than other modalities. In other words, PET can examine the fundamental biological function of a disease in its early stages, in many cases, before symptoms occur" (Crozer-Keystone Health System 2001, p. 1). My own experience with PET scanning is given in Chapter 3.

8. Gleevec and Herceptin are examples of a new class of anticancer drugs that disrupt the molecular functioning of cancer cells. Gleevec (imatinib mesylate) disrupts the activity of an oncogenic fusion gene, bcr-abl, which

causes chronic myeloid leukemia (CML). Because CML is precipitated from one genetic lesion, it is particularly apt for targeted therapies. Initial studies of Gleevec produced remarkable responses in CML patients. There is some evidence that Gleevec is an effective treatment in gastrointestinal stromal sarcoma (GIST) as well as Kaposi's sarcoma. See Moses and Fruh (2002) and Hauser (2002), and O'Dwyer and Druker (2000). Like Gleevec, Herceptin (Trastuzumab), targets an oncogene, HER2 (human epidermal growth-factor, receptor2), which is overexpressed in breast cancer. Studies have indicated that Herceptin is well tolerated and produces durable tumor responses. See Leyland-Jones (2002).

9. In the words of a report published by the Institute of Medicine (2001), there are increasing indications of a growing "quality chasm" in medical care. Despite increased investment in medical technology, there is a large literature that documents the difficulties that medical institutions have in producing health. The shortcomings are seen in the experience of patients in (a) small care units, (b) in larger organizations, and (c) with bureaucracies that form policies, write regulations, exact payments. These institutional shortcomings and consequent quality deficits have in turn arguably dehumanized medicine. See also Newhouse (2002) and Berwick (2002). Other works that speak to the issue of confidence in health care include Pellegrino and Thomasma (1988); Cassell (1991); Friedson (1989); Veatch (1991); and Waitzkin (1991).

10. For more information on how patients and physicians can deal with diagnostic uncertainty, see Franklin (1983). For more details on rumination see Nolen-Hoeksema (2000) and Lyubomirsky and Nolen-Hoeksema (1995).

CHAPTER TWO:
HARMONIZING THE BUSH AT THE CANCER CENTER

1. Indolent low-grade follicular B-cell lymphoma remains, for the most part, an incurable disease. Colombat et al (2001) writes that the "optimal treatment of advanced-stage NHL is yet to be determined. In patients with low tumor burden and without adverse prognostic factors, retrospective analysis and prospective studies have shown that postponing treatment until progression has no negative influence on survival. Nevertheless, almost all patients will experience disease progression and ultimately die of their disease" (p. 101). The Physician Data Query (PDQ) of the National Cancer Institute for adult NHL treatment sets the median NHL survival at ten years. Other studies that assess NHL survival include Yuen, Kamel,

and Halpern et al. (1995); Armitage (1993); and Bastion, Sebban, and Berger et al. (1997).

2. See Passmore (1968); Putnam (1992); and Austin (1961).

3. There is a long-standing debate in both sociology and anthropology about rationality. Scholars take three stances on rationality. There are the universalists, who use logic and scientific method to make judgments about beliefs and practices. For them science and logic are prior to other systems of beliefs. There are the relativists, who take varying positions on the autonomy of belief systems. Finally, there are the phenomenologists, who argue for a multiplicity of realities as a way to bridge the considerable conceptual gaps forged by universalists and relativists. See Evans-Pritchard (1937); Wilson (1970); Sperber (1985); Geertz (1984); Jackson (1996, 1998); and Stoller (1998).

4. Contemporary physicians seem to take several stances toward medical skepticism. Some are concerned that given the unprecedented growth of medical knowledge and time constraints, physicians have neither the time nor the willingness to adequately ponder diagnostic variables or treatment decisions. Mark J. DiNubile (2000) considers skepticism a lost clinical art:

> In our modern era of unprecedented scientific growth, where significant biomedical advancements are daily occurrences, it appears that contemporary physicians have become more willing to accept the "latest and greatest" without careful scrutiny. We as a profession seem more preoccupied with sins of omission and less concerned about errors of commission. This new trend routinely bucks our conservative traditions; after all, the first rule of medicine is not "to do good" but emphatically "to do no harm." The current predominant modus operandi reverses these priorities in many cases, often to the patient's detriment. (p. 513)

Physicians are also skeptical of alternative medicine, which has grown by leaps and bounds in the recent past. Former surgeon general C. Everett Koop (2002) has been concerned about how the rapid growth of alternative medicines for AIDS and for tobacco addiction has precipitated health problems. Harlan (2001) advocates the extension of clinical trial methodologies, which are rigorous, to the evaluation of what he calls "complementary and alternative medicine modalities." Taking a more open-ended stance, Martin (2001) suggests that an overly conservative skepticism may retard medical progress:

The popularity of complementary and alternative treatments has grown enormously in recent years. Physicians must understand what therapies our patients are using and how these therapies work. We must ask if these therapies interact with medicines we prescribe. We must recognize that medical care is both a science, and a connection between patient and healer. And we must be open to the likelihood that, as in the past, some therapies that are now considered alternative will be standard practice in the future. (p. 11)

5. There has been much discussion of divination in ethnographic reports on societies in West and Central Africa. Among the most celebrated texts are Adler and Zempleni (1972) on the Moundang of Chad, Bascom (1994) on the Yoruba of Nigeria, and Peek's collection on African divination systems (1991). Shaw (2002) has produced a fine ethnography that describes how divination, among other practices, shapes memory and contours the historical imagination of the Temne of Sierra Leone. Shaw claims, quite rightly, that by linking present and past, most West African divination systems help to forge an atmosphere of completeness, harmony, and continuity. Beyond these practices of harmonization, as Shaw astutely observes, the practice also embodies uncertainty and danger. Divination

> is concerned with danger. Such crises as sudden death, problematic childbirth, illness, and collapsing granaries erupt above and beyond "ordinary" predicaments demanding action that departs from that of everyday practice. But an exploration of Temne divination entails a broader focus than that on the crises precipitating the consultation of diviners; it also requires attention to certain dangers perceived in the very nature of divination itself. These dangers are mapped within divination techniques, experienced during diviners' initiatory visions, and represented as inherent in the persons of diviners themselves. (p. 5)

Shaw's broad approach to West African divination has striking parallels to the diagnostic processes central to Western medical practice. In times of physical crisis, we seek out physicians, who, in order to make a diagnosis, order diagnostic tests, most of which entail some ritual elements as well as some degree of risk. Tests are called "procedures" and are filled with ritualistic preparations—fasts, premedication, qualifying blood work, ingestion of barium. The iodine administered during a contrast CAT scan, after all, can produce a fatal allergic reaction.

6. Much has been written about the advisability of certain medical screening tests, especially procedures used to detect prostate and breast cancer. Despite much discussion about the poor record of PSA (prostate-specific antigen) screening tests, recent data suggests that overdiagnosis of prostate cancer in PSA tests is not as prevalent as expected (see Etzioni et. al. 2002 and Slovin 2002). In the case of breast cancer, much has been made of the efficacy of mammograms. In September 2001 the Canadian National Breast Cancer Screening Study showed that combining mammography, self-examination, and physician examination did not reduce the death rate from the disease for women in their forties as compared with self and physician examination alone (see Miller, To, Baines, and Wall 2002). This finding flies in the face of received medical wisdom, which means that most physicians continue to recommend regularly scheduled mammograms for women over forty. Conflicting findings, which are common in science and in medicine, lead to diagnostic doubt.

7. American optimism is a folk category in the culture of the United States. Many Americans believe that it is ongoing optimism—the spirit of "can do"—that has made America great. In a 2002 book, *The American Paradox*, David Myers considers the eroding civility of contemporary American social life, but suggests a shift toward optimism in both public forums and private conversations. The September 11 terrorist attacks have challenged American optimism, but according to most reports, terrorism hasn't dampened the American penchant for optimism. Although terrorism has reduced American consumer confidence, Americans are optimistic that the United States will win the war on terrorism. "Along with the surge in patriotism, our tracking measures of the overall mood of the nation reflect Americans' characteristic optimism in the face of adversity." See Wirthlin (2001), Page (2002), and American Association of Retired People Research Group (2002).

8. Given the militaristic metaphors that are utilized to categorize the "war" on cancer, it is not uncommon for people to think of malignant cells as alien invaders, as not part of the body, or to use A. David Napier's (2003) phrase, as "non-self." Despite this widespread notion, cancer is something that the body—your body—produces. As stated by Frank (1991), "Cancer is not some entity separate from yourself. . . . Most people opt for the tumor-as-alien. At the extreme is Ronald Reagan's well-known statement about his

cancer. 'I don't have cancer. I had something inside of me that had cancer in it, and it was removed,' sums up this unwillingness to understand cancer as part of yourself" (p. 84).

9. Page (2002).

10. See Schulz, Bookwald, Scherer, Knapp, and Williamson (1996).

11. Frank (1995, 46–48).

12. Indolent NHL is a highly treatable disease. Many patients respond well to chemotherapy and immunotherapy and achieve a complete response. Initial remission may—or may not—be of long duration. When disease progression recurs, patients undergo new treatments, which may include monoclonal antibodies, bone marrow, and/or stem cell replacements. In more advanced stages of the disease, periods between remission and disease progression become shorter and shorter. As it now stands, in its advanced stages, NHL is incurable. See Press (2000), Colombat et al. (2001), and Levine (2001).

13. For ethnographic information on Songhay social relations see Olivier de Sardan (1982, 1984), Rouch (1989), Sidikou (1974), and Stoller (1989a, 1989b, 1995). There is a vast literature in social psychology on sources on individualism and collectivism. Among the most prominent titles include Hofstede (1980) and Triandis (1995), both of which are attempts to measure the degree of individualism and collectivism in society. These binary opposites, however useful in comparing and contrasting societies, can lead to oversimplification and essentialism, especially in the contemporary climate of what Mark Taylor (2002) has termed "network culture," in which increasing technological sophistication has greatly eroded cultural distance and difference. Many of these distinctions, though certainly not all of them, get mixed together in a maze of complex systems, which undermine the relevance and suitability of binary opposites.

14. There are many studies on the relation of cancer to the onset of depression. See McDaniel et al. (1995), Sheard and Maguire (1999), Barraclough (1998), Miller (2002), and Lan Ly (2002).

CHAPTER THREE: TREATMENT

1. There is a large literature on social support in social psychology and in gerontology. Some of the more important studies include: Krause (1990), Rodin (1986), Mirowski (1995), and Kahn and Antonucci (1980).

2. See Cole (2001) and Shaw (2002) for fine ethnographic studies of divination in African societies. Cole's study probed memory and some divinatory practices in Madagascar. Shaw considers divination and social memory in Sierra Leone.

3. See Rouch (1989).

4. See Rouch (1989), Stoller (1989b; 1998), and Stoller and Olkes (1987).

5. There has been a spate of works on technology and the increased velocity of social life in the contemporary world. There is also an emerging literature on social complexity. Some of these works attempt to use the insights of cognitive science to refine social and cultural analysis (Bloch 1998; Turner 2002). Taylor (2002) argues that contemporary social theory, based upon modernity's grid-like binary oppositions, is ill equipped to explain, let alone comprehend, what has become what he calls "network" culture. Taylor writes: "For more than three decades, Foucault's constructivism, Derrida's deconstruction, and Baudrillard's account of simulacra have combined to form rich resources from which to assess various social and cultural developments. However, as we move into a new era, the limitations of these lines of analysis are becoming obvious. The creative possibilities of network culture cannot be understood unless new interpretive trajectories are fashioned" (p. 72). See also Castells (1996, 1997, 1998) on the complexity of social and culture systems.

6. There are many proverbs among the Songhay people that underscore the need to be well prepared for any task one might undertake. Several of the most frequently used of these include: (1) *Hala fakey ga boro zaarey, a si du hangan* (When you are thrown by a donkey, you cannot stop your fall by catching the donkey's ear); (2) *Me ra hari si denjii wi* (One mouthful of water will not douse a fire); and (3) *Ni bon bay za borey mana ni bay* (Know yourself before others get to know you). As the first proverb suggests, no matter a person's athletic skill, if he or she doesn't know how to ride a donkey, the beast of burden will throw him or her, and the donkey's ear is much too small to stop the fall. The second proverb urges proper preparation. If you only have one mouthful of water, your attempts to put out the fire will be futile. The third proverb is central to the apprenticeship of sorcerers and griots. For them, you must master yourself before you can let others know what you know.

7. See Stoller (1989b, 121–22).

8. See Franklin (1983) and Barraclough (1998).

9. The neurological effects of vincristine are widely reported. See Naumann et al. (2001), Haim et al. (1994), and Balis and Poplack (1989).

CHAPTER FOUR: REMISSIONING LIFE

1. For a fine presentation on the quandaries of remission, see Frank (1995).

2. There are tens of thousands of cancer support groups throughout the world. A quick check on the Internet suggests that cancer centers, large and small, urban and rural, all sponsor and recommend that cancer patients join a support group. The goals of support groups are uniform. Based on extensive research by social psychologists like Krause (1990), it is known that participation in support groups decreases patient alienation, reduces patient anxiety, increases the patient's comprehension of cancer, and diminishes feelings of isolation and hopelessness. There are several kinds of support groups. Some focus on education. These emphasize health-enhancing behaviors and uncover misconceptions and myths about cancer. There are support groups that focus on coping skills, including resources in alternative medicine. There are also support groups that become psychological forums that help patients to adjust to their circumstances. See also Holland (1982); Holland and Lewis (2000); and Lauria, Stearns, and Hermann (2001).

3. See Stoller and Olkes (1987).

4. See Frank (1995).

CHAPTER FIVE:
BEARING WITNESS ON THE WINGS OF THE WIND

1. See Sontag (1978), Frank (1991, 1995), and Alsop (1973).

2. The notion of the "wings of the wind" is borrowed from the Dogon people of Mali, when they refer to the Sigui ceremonies, held every sixty years and performed once a year for seven years. The Sigui celebrates, among other things, the origin of death and of speech. When the Sigui begins, the drums beat and the Dogon sing: "The Sigui takes off on the wings of the wind." See Rouch (1978, 17–18).

References

Adler, Alfred, and Andras Zempleni. 1972. *Le baton de l'aveugle: Divination, maladie et Pouvoir chez les Moundang du Tchad.* Paris: Hermann.

Ainsworth-Vaughn, Nancy. 1998. *Claiming Power in Doctor-Patient Talk.* New York: Oxford University Press.

Alsop, Stuart. 1973. *Stay of Execution.* Philadelphia: Lippincott.

American Association of Retired People Research Group. 2002. Money and the American Family. *Modern Maturity,* May.

Andrews, Lynn V. 1981. *Medicine Woman.* San Francisco: Harper and Row.

Armitage, James O. 1993. Treatment of Non-Hodgkin's Lymphoma. *New England Journal of Medicine* 328, no. 14:1023–1030.

Austin, J. L. 1961. *Philosophical Papers.* Oxford: Clarendon Press.

Balis, F. M., and D. G. Poplack. 1989. Central Nervous System Pharmacology of Antileukemic Drugs. *American Journal of Pediatric Hematology and Oncology* 11, no. 1:74–86.

Barraclough, B. 1998. *Cancer and Emotion: A Practical Guide to Psycho-Oncology.* 3d ed. Chichester, U.K.: John Wiley.

Barclay, Laurie. 2002a. Controversy Rages over Breast Cancer Screening. *Medscape Medical News,* 2 September 2003.

———. 2002b. Controversy Rages Over Breast Cancer Screening: An Interview with Newsmaker Michael Baum, MD. *Medscape Medical News,* 3 September 2002.

Bascom, William. 1994. *Ifa Divination: Communication between Gods and Men in West Africa*. Bloomington: Indiana University Press.

Bastion, Y., C. Sebban, and F. Berger et al. 1997. Incidence, Predictive Factors and Outcomes of Lymphoma Transformation in Follicular Lymphoma Patients. *Journal of Clinical Oncology* 15, no. 4:1587–1594.

Berwick, Donald M. 2002. A User's Manual for the IOM's Quality Chasm Report. *Health Affairs* 21, no. 3:80–90.

Bloch, Maurice. 1998. *How We Think They Think*. Boulder, Colo.: Westview Press.

Cassell, Eric J. 1991. *The Nature of Suffering and the Goals of Medicine*. New York: Oxford University Press.

Castells, Manuel. 1996. *The Rise of Network Society*. Cambridge, Mass: Blackwell.

———. 1997. *The Power of Identity*. Cambridge, Mass: Blackwell.

———. 1998. *End of the Millennium*. Cambridge, Mass: Blackwell.

Cole, Jennifer. 2001. *Forget Colonialism?: Sacrifice and the Art of Memory in Madagascar*. Berkeley and Los Angeles: University of California Press.

Crozer-Keystone Health System. 2001. Positron Emission Tomography. Informational brochure.

Colombat, Phillipe et al. 2001. Rituximab (anti CD20 monoclonal antibody) as Single First-Line Therapy for Patients with Follicular Lymphoma with a Low Tumor Burden: Clinical and Molecular Evaluation. *Blood* 97, no. 1:101–106.

Dewey, John. 1980. *The Quest for Certainty*. New York: Minton, Balch, 1929. Reprint, New York: Perigree Books.

DiNubile, Mark J. 2000. Skepticism: A Lost Clinical Art. *Clinical Infectious Diseases* 31:513–518.

Drescher, Fran. 2002. *Cancer Schmancer*. New York: Warner Books.

Etzioni, Ruth et.al. 2002. Overdiagnosis Due to Prostate-Specific Antigen Screening: Lessons from US Prostate Cancer Incidence Trends. *Journal of the National Cancer Institute* 94:981–990.

Evans-Pritchard, E. E. 1976. *Witchcraft, Oracles and Magic among the Azande*. Oxford: Clarendon Press, 1937. Reprint, Oxford: Clarendon Press.

Fisher, Sue. 1986. *In the Patient's Best Interest: Women and the Politics of Medical Decisions.* New Brunswick, N.J.: Rutgers University Press.

Fisher, Sue, and Alexandra Todd, eds. 1993. *The Social Organization of Doctor-Patient Communication.* 2d ed. Norwood, N.J.: Ablex.

Frank, Arthur. 1991. *At the Will of the Body.* Boston: Houghton Mifflin.

————. 1995. *The Wounded Storyteller: Body, Illness and Ethics.* Chicago: University of Chicago Press.

Franklin, Jon. 1983. *Not Quite a Miracle: Brain Surgeons and Their Patients on the Frontier of Medicine.* Garden City, N.J.: Doubleday.

Friedson, Eliot. 1989. *Medical Work in America: Essays on Health Care.* New Haven, Conn.: Yale University Press.

Geertz, Clifford. 1984. Anti Anti-relativism. *American Anthropologist* 86, no. 2:263–278.

Haim N., R. Epelbaum, and M. Ben-Shahar. 1994. Full Dose Vincristine (without 2-mg Dose Limit) in the Treatment of Lymphomas. *Cancer* 73:2515–2519.

Harlan, William. 2001. New Opportunities and Proven Approaches in Complementary and Alternative Medicine at the National Institutes of Health. *Journal of Alternative and Complementary Medicine* 7, no. 6:53–60.

Hofstede, Geert. 1980. *Culture's Consequences: International Differences in Work-Related Values.* Beverly Hills, Calif.: Sage.

Holland, Jimmie. 1982. *Current Concepts in Psychosocial Oncology.* New York: Memorial Sloan-Kettering.

Holland, Jimmie C., and Sheldon Lewis. 2000. *The Human Side of Cancer: Living with Hope, Coping with Uncertainty.* New York: Harper-Collins.

Hussar, Daniel A. 2001. New Drugs of 2001. *Journal of the American Pharmaceutical Association* 42, no. 3:227–260.

Institute of Medicine. 2001. *Crossing the Quality Chasm: A New Health System for the Twenty-first Century.* Washington, D.C.: National Academy Press.

Jackson, Michael, ed. 1996. *Things As They Are: New Directions in Phenomenological Anthropology.* Bloomington: Indiana University Press.

Jackson, Michael. 1998. *Minima Ethnographica.* Chicago: University of Chicago Press.

Kahn, R. L., and L. C. Antonucci. 1980. Convoys over the Life Course: Attachment, Roles and Social Support. In *Life-span Development and Behavior*. Vol. 3, ed. by P. B. Baltes and O. G. Brim, 254–286. New York: Academic Press.

Koop, C. Everett. 2002. The Future of Medicine. *Science* 295:233.

Krause, N. 1990. Perceived Health Problems, Formal/Informal Support and Life Satisfaction among Older Adults. *Journal of Gerontology: Social Sciences* 45:193–205.

Lan Ly, K. 2002. Depression in Advanced Disease: A Systematic Review. Part 1: Prevalence and Case Finding. *Palliative Medicine* 16:81–98.

Lauria, Marie, Naomi Stearns, and Joan Hermann. 2001. *Social Work in Oncology: Supporting Survivors, Families and Caregivers*. New York: American Cancer Society.

Levine, Alexandra. 2001. Revisiting and Revising Therapeutic Strategies for Lymphoma. Reportage. In Papers read at the European Cancer Conference, ECCO 11, Lisbon, Portugal, 21 October.

Leyland-Jones, B. 2002. Targeting HER2: Hopes and Realities. *Lancet Oncology* 3:137–144.

Lyubomirksy, Sonja, and Susan Noel-Hoeksema. 1995. Effects of Self-Focused Rumination on Negative Thinking and Interpersonal Problem Solving. *Journal of Personality and Aging* 69, no. 1:176–190.

Martin, Joseph B. 2001. Historical and Professional Perspectives on Complementary and Alternative Medicine with a Particular Emphasis on Rediscovering and Embracing Complementary and Alternative Medicine in Contemporary Western Society. *Journal of Alternative and Complementary Medicine* 7, no. 6:11–19.

McDaniel, J. S. et.al. 1995. Depression in Patients with Cancer: Diagnosis, Biology and Treatment. *Archives of General Psychiatry* 52:89–99.

Miller, A. B., T. To, C. J. Baines, and C. Wall. 2002. The Canadian National Breast Screening Study-1: Breast Cancer Mortality after Eleven to Sixteen Years of Follow-up; A Randomized Screening Trial of Mammography in Women Ages Forty to Forty-nine Years. *Annals of Internal Medicine* 137, no. 5:305–312.

Miller, Douglas K. 2002. Psychosocial-Spiritual Correlates of Death Distress in Patients with Life-Threatening Medical Conditions. *Palliative Medicine* 16, no. 4:331–338.

Mirowski, J. 1995. Age and the Sense of Control. *Social Psychology Quarterly* 58, no. 1:31–34.

Moses, Ashlee W., and Klaus Fruh. 2002. Karposi's Sarcoma-Associated Herpesvirus-induced Upregulation of the c-kit Proto Oncogene, as Identified by Gene Expression Profiling, Is Essential for the Transformation of Endothelial Cells. *Journal of Virology* 76, no. 16:8393–8399.

Myers, David G. 2002. *The American Paradox: Spiritual Hunger in the Age of Plenty.* New Haven, Conn.: Yale University Press.

Napier, A. David. 2003. *The Age of Immunology.* Chicago: University of Chicago Press.

National Cancer Institute. 2002. *PDQ Adult Non-Hodgkin's Lymphoma.* Washington, D.C.: U.S. Government Printing Office.

Naumann, Ralph, Johannes Mohm, Ulrike Reuner, Frank Kroschinsky, Bernd Rautenstrass, and Gerhard Ehninger. 2001. Early Recognition of Hereditary and Sensory Neuropathy Type 1 Can Avoid Life-threatening Vincristine Neurotoxicity. *British Journal of Haemotology* 111, no. 2:323–326.

Newhouse, Jack. 2002. Why Is There a Quality Chasm? *Health Affairs* 21, no. 4:13–25.

Nolen-Hoeksema, Susan. 2000. The Role of Rumination in Depressive Disorders and Mixed Anxiety/Depressive Symptoms. *Journal of Abnormal Psychology* 109, no. 3:504–512.

O'Dwyer, M. E., and B. J. Druker. 2000. ST1571: A BCR-ABL TK Inhibitor for the Treatment of CML. *Lancet Oncology* 1:207–211.

Olivier de Sardan, Jean-Pierre. 1982. *Concepts et conceptions Zarma-Songhay.* Paris: Nubia.

———. 1984. *Sociétés Songay-Zarma.* Paris: Karthala.

Page, Clarence. 2002. American Optimism Surges Despite Tragedy, Heartache. *Salt Lake Tribune,* 10 January.

Passmore, John. 1968. *Hume's Intentions.* New York: Basic Books.

Peek, Philip M., ed. 1991. *African Divination Systems: Ways of Knowing.* Bloomington: Indiana University Press.

Pellegrino, Edmund D., and David C. Thomasma. 1988. *For the Patient's Good: The Restoration of Beneficence in Health Care.* New York: Oxford University Press.

Press, Oliver W. 2000. Emerging Immunotherapies for Non-Hodgkin Lymphomas: The Tortoise Approaches the Finish Line. *Annals of Internal Medicine* 132:916–918.

Putnam, Hilary. 1992. *Renewing Philosophy.* Cambridge, Mass.: Harvard University Press.

Rodin, Judith. 1986. Aging and Health: Effects of the Sense of Control. *Sciences* 23:1271–1276.

Rouch, Jean. 1978. Le renard fou et le maitre pale. In *Systèmes des signes: Textes réunis En hommage à Germaine Dieterlen,* 3–24. Paris: Hermann.

Rouch, Jean. 1989. *La religion et la magie Songhay.* 2d ed. Brussels: Free University Press.

Schultz, Richard, Jamila Bookwald, Michael Scherer, Judith Knapp, and Gail M. Williamsom. 1996. Pessimism, Age and Cancer Mortality. *Psychology and Aging* 11, no. 2:304–309

Seligman, Martin J. 1991. *Learned Optimism.* New York: Knopf.

Shaw, Rosalind. 2002. *Memories of the Slave Trade: Ritual and the Historical Imagination in Sierra Leone.* Chicago: University of Chicago Press.

Sheard, T., and P. Maguire. 1999. The Effect of Psychological Interventions on Anxiety and Depression in Cancer Patients: Results of Two Meta-analyses. *British Journal of Cancer* 80:1770–1780.

Shuy, Roger. 1993. Three Types of Interference to an Effective Exchange of Information in the Medical Interview. In *The Social Organization of Doctor-Patient Communication,* ed. by Alexandra Dundas Todd and Sue Fisher, 189–202. 2d ed. Norwood, N.J.: Ablex.

Sidikou, Harouna. 1974. *Sendentarité et mobilité entre Niger et Zagret.* Etudes Nigeriennes no. 34. Niamey: Université de Niamey.

Slovin, Susan. 2002. Biochemical Relapse in Prostate Cancer: Is PSA Promoting Stress and Anxiety? *Medscape Hematology-Oncology e-Journal* 5, no. 4: 1–6.

Sontag, Susan. 1978. *Illness as Metaphor.* New York: Farrar, Strauss and Giroux.

Sperber, Dan. 1985. *On Anthropological Knowledge*. Cambridge, U.K.: Cambridge University Press.

Stoller, Paul. 1989a. *Fusion of the Worlds: An Ethnography of Possession among the Songhay of Niger*. Chicago: University of Chicago Press.

————. 1989b. *The Taste of Ethnographic Things: The Senses in Anthropology*. Philadelphia: University of Pennsylvania Press.

————. 1995. *Embodying Colonial Memories: Spirit Possession, Power and the Hauka in West Africa*. New York: Routledge.

————. 1997. *Sensuous Scholarship*. Philadelphia: University of Pennsylvania Press.

————. 1998. Rationality. In *Critical Terms in Religious Studies*, ed. by Mark C. Taylor, 239–256. Chicago: University of Chicago Press.

Stoller, Paul, and Cheryl Olkes. 1987. *In Sorcery's Shadow: A Memoir of Apprenticeship among the Songhay of Niger*. Chicago: University of Chicago Press.

Taylor, Mark C. 2002. *The Moment of Complexity: The Emergence of Network Culture*. Chicago: University of Chicago Press.

Triandis, Harry. 1995. *Individualism and Collectivism*. Boulder, Colo.: Westview Press.

Turner, Stephen P. 2002. *Brains/Practices/Relativism: Social Theory after Cognitive Science*. Chicago: University of Chicago Press.

Turner, Victor. 1969. *The Ritual Process: Structure and Anti-structure*. Ithaca, N.Y.: Cornell University Press.

Veatch, Robert M. 1991. *The Patient-Physician Relation: The Patient as Partner, Part 2*. Bloomington: Indiana University Press.

Waitzkin, Howard. 1991. *Politics of Medical Encounters: How Patients and Doctors Deal with Social Problems*. New Haven, Conn.: Yale University Press.

Wilson, Bryan R., ed. 1970. *Rationality*. Evanston, Ill.: Harper and Row.

Wirthlin, Richard. 2001. America Responds. *Wirthlin Report* 11, no. 10:1–4.

Yuen, A. R., D. W. Kamel, and J. Halpern et al. 1995. Long-Term Survival after Histological Transformation of Low-Grade Follicular Lymphoma. *Journal of Clinical Oncology* 13, no. 7:1721–1733.

Author's Note

The memoir is a challenging literary form. Memoirists always run the risk of making their works either too personal or not personal enough. How much personal detail should you include? How important is it to reinforce the drama, if any exists, of the narrative? Are the details of your life interesting enough to be told? If so, are the lessons of your lived experience instructive to others?

Because of the technical, literary, and emotional challenges of writing *Stranger in the Village of the Sick*, I asked many friends and colleagues for their help. For their constructive and encouraging comments I am deeply indebted to Helen Berger, John Chernoff, Steven Dickter, Janice Dickter, Susan DiGiacomo, Jean-Paul Dumont, Eli Dumont, David Grossman, A. David Napier, Patricia Smith, and John Wolfe. Their incisive comments, some about the technical particularities of medicine, some about the textual particularities of the memoir, have sharpened the accuracy of the book's content and have refined its structure. With her characteristic thoroughness, Jasmin Tahmaseb McConatha read and reread all the drafts of *Stranger in the Village of the Sick*. If my experiences in the worlds of sorcery and cancer have succeeded in resonating with a diverse audience, it is due in large measure to her commitment and diligence.

As readers may have noticed, I have tried to obscure the identity of the facility where I received medical treatment. I also changed the names of the physicians and nurses who diagnosed my lymphoma and treated me for it. I used pseudonyms to protect the privacy of these dedicated professionals. The use of pseudonyms in no way reflects a negative assessment of their professionalism or clinical capacities. Their knowledge of cutting-edge cancer treatments and their ability to use that knowledge in creative ways has, in effect, prolonged my life and made me a more reflective person. These are debts that cannot be fully repaid. As always, the wisdom of Adamu Jenitongo has guided me in fruitful directions. This book is a small token of my gratitude to him. Finally, I am grateful to the scores of cancer patients I have met. In moments of great anxiety and substantial pain, they taught me the meaning of the word *dignity*.

Index